D1519447

CONTROL OF PAIN AND OTHER SYMPTOMS IN CANCER PATIENTS

THE CANCER SERIES

Jan Vincents Johannessen, Series Editor

In Preparation

CONTROL OF PAIN AND OTHER SYMPTOMS IN CANCER PATIENTS

Tor Inge Tønnessen

The Norwegian Radium Hospital,
Montebello, Oslo 3, Norway

●HEMISPHERE PUBLISHING CORPORATION
A member of the Taylor & Francis Group
New York   Washington   Philadelphia   London

CONTROL OF PAIN AND OTHER SYMPTOMS IN CANCER PATIENTS

1 2 3 4 5 6 7 8 9 0   E B E B   9 8 7 6 5 4 3 2 1 0 9

This book was set in Palacio type by Hemisphere Publishing Corporation. The editors were Mary Prescott and John P. Rowan; the designer was Sharon Martin DePass; the production supervisor was Peggy M. Rote; and the typesetter was Shirley J. McNett. Allison Olsen translated the text from the Norwegian.
Cover design by Renee Winfield.
This book was originally published as *Smerter og andre symptomer hos kreftpasienter,* by Universitetsforlaget AS.

Library of Congress Cataloging-in-Publication Data

Tønnessen, Tor Inge.
  Control of pain and other symptoms in cancer patients / Tor Inge Tønnessen.
  p. cm. (The Cancer series)

    1. Cancer—Palliative treatment. 2. Cancer pain—Treatment.
  I. Title. II. Series: Cancer series (New York, N.Y.)
    [DNLM: 1. Neoplasms—therapy. 2. Pain—therapy.   QZ 266 T666c]
  RC271.P33T66   1989
  616.99'40472—dc20
  DNLM/DLC
  for Library of Congress   89-19873
  ISBN 0-89116-868-0   CIP
  ISSN 1043-9439

Contents

Foreword

Contrary to common belief, cancer pain is not an inevitable part of cancer. The right drug in the right dose at the right time can control more than 80 percent of cancer pain. A scientifically valid and relatively inexpensive method already exists to treat cancer pain.

Despite this, cancer pain relief is often not offered. The World Health Organization (WHO) estimates that some 3.5 million people suffer daily worldwide, and many cancer patients suffer unnecessarily from severe pain with little or no relief, although they are treated for their tumor. Even for the terminally ill, cancer pain is unrelieved.

In the developed countries, at present, two thirds of the cancer patients will die of their disease. In the developing countries, where more than half of the world's cancer patients live, the majority of them are incurable at the time of diagnosis. Relief of cancer pain and other symptoms is most often the only humane alternative one can offer to the patients. Knowledge already exists on the relief of major symptoms of cancer patients. Our resources, strategies, and priorities in the care of cancer patients should be reshuffled to ensure that major symptoms of cancer patients are adequately relieved.

Two major concerns of cancer patients and their families are (1) whether the patient will have a lot of pain and (2) whether the patient will die alone. Unrelieved pain is still a major symptom in terminally ill cancer patients. With the help of the knowledge presented in this book, most pain could be controlled, and families, nurses, and doctors could feel confident in being able to handle the major symptoms, thus motivating them to be present. Up to now, palliative care of the patient has been neglected at the expense of therapy.

Tor Inge Tønnessen, the author of this book, works at the Radium Hospitalet in Norway, and it is significant that, again, the largest cancer hospital in Scandinavia has taken the lead.

In this concise, logical, and didactic book, Dr. Tønnessen shows how pain and other cancer symptoms can be controlled and clearly defines the existing knowledge. Dr. Tønnessen's work, together with the WHO monograph "Cancer Pain Relief," should be widely used by doctors, nurses, and other health care providers to implement adequate symptom relief of cancer patients everywhere, thus improving their quality of life.

JAN STJERNEWÄRD, M.D.
Chief, Cancer Unit
World Health Organization

Preface

Interest in the control of pain and other symptoms has increased enormously in recent years. Palliation and the care of patients with a poor life expectancy have become a focus of attention, both in medical circles and in the media. Interdisciplinary counseling groups have been set up at a number of hospitals and hospices to help and advise patients, their families, and health professionals on the relief of symptoms and the care of seriously ill and dying people. Courses and conferences on the subject are also becoming common.

But although so much progress has been made in palliative medicine, a large number of health professionals are still not familiar with this field. Thousands of patients suffer unnecessarily from their symptoms. The widespread lack of knowledge about pain relief makes it essential to collect and systematically organize the information and experience we have in this area, and the fact that the first edition of the book has already been sold out shows how much this information is needed. The response to the first edition was very positive, and in the preparation of this new English language edition I have tried to take into account the negative as well as the positive criticism.

The book is written for physicians, medical students, nurses, and student nurses. It is divided into three main parts: *understanding* of pain, *methods* for treating pain and other symptoms, and *practical applications* of the principles of treatment. Part I deals with background knowledge—anatomy and physiology, assessment of pain, and principles of treatment.

Part II describes analgesics and other drugs used in pain and other symptomatic therapy. (In the text, all drugs are referred to by their generic names only. In Appendix 1 both generic names and trade names are given.) Part II also describes other methods of treating these symptoms, including nerve blocks, neurosurgery, palliative surgery, radiotherapy, chemotherapy, and hormone therapy. Part III describes how the methods of treatment can be carried out and integrated in everyday clinical work, and this part of the book can be read independently. Each chapter is designed to be intelligible when read on its own, so the reader will find a number of repetitions. A short and practical introduction to symptom control can be obtained by reading Chapters 2, 3, 10, 11, and 12. The remaining chapters contain the background information necessary for making a thorough assessment and treatment plan for each patient. A thorough description of psychic reactions to serious illness and death is beyond the scope of this book.

The list of contents has been given in detail to facilitate easy reference. The English version has been updated and adapted to conditions in the United States.

My grateful thanks go to the following people, who read parts of the manuscript and gave me help and advice: Professor Harald Breivik, the National Hospital; Dr. Steinar Bjørgo, the Norwegian Radium Hospital; Dr. Kjell Magne Tveit, the Norwegian Radium Hospital; and Dr. Ellen Jørum, University of Oslo. I should also like to thank Jon Håvard Loge of the Norwegian University Press for his help and cooperation.

Last of all, Åsa, Sven Richard, and Cecilia deserve special thanks for representing the best possible prophylaxis against the "burnout syndrome."

TOR INGE TØNNESSEN

Introduction

Most people are afraid of cancer. Almost everyone has a friend or relative who has suffered a great deal of pain from this frightening disease. One can hardly open a newspaper without reading that someone has died "after a long and painful illness." Cancer is therefore justifiably associated in most people's minds with pain and suffering. Far too many people have suffered so much at the end of their lives that it has affected their contact with their families and surroundings.

Everyone is afraid of pain. Surveys show that a great many people worry about the possibility of dying painfully, and that they are more afraid of this than of death itself.

More than half of the patients who die of cancer will experience severe pain during their illness. A quarter of them will have moderate or mild pain, and the remaining quarter of them will not experience any pain at all. Thousands of people are thus suffering night and day from one of the worst experiences a human being can go through.

Health professionals are often in contact with these people and their suffering, and considering the extent of the problem, one would assume that medical science has come a long way toward solving it. Fortunately it has. Good tools have been developed to handle pain, but paradoxically enough, there are far too many who are not able to use them properly. Several surveys have revealed a great deal of ignorance among medical personnel about the use of painkilling drugs in chronic diseases. The teaching of medical students has been very inadequate in this respect, and even experienced physicians often know surprisingly little about it.

Interest in the problem of pain has increased steadily during the last 10 to 20 years. Great progress has been made in the English-speaking countries and in Scandinavia, and the improvement in knowledge is gradually spreading to the rest of the world. Surveys have shown that more than 90% of patients obtain substantial relief from pain if given proper treatment, and this development can be counted as a very great achievement in modern medicine.

Acute pain with an obvious etiology and a good prognosis, like a broken leg, is a completely different experience from chronic pain. Acute pain is easier to tolerate, even when it is more intense, than chronic pain. Patients with cancer know that the pain will probably get worse, and they can see no solution. They have no control over the pain, and this makes them feel helpless. The pain seems meaningless. This kind of pain almost always gives rise to depression and anxiety, which in turn aggravate the pain, and the patient is caught in a vicious circle.

People with severe chronic pain are dominated by it; it occupies their thoughts, destroys their concentration, and takes all their energy. The pain is no longer a symptom of a disease process, it is the person's main problem. We should therefore take it seriously when the patient asks for help. We should bring the same therapeutic enthusiasm to relieving the symptoms that we devote to seeking a remission to the disease, even when we know that the patient cannot be cured.

Other symptoms besides pain also require professional diagnosis and treatment. Palliation has been a neglected area of medical practice and research for far too long. Using relatively simple methods, we can give patients the help they need to be able to live with and cope with their disease for a short or long period. Palliative treatment is an interesting field in which a great many advances have recently been made.

The first phase of cancer usually involves active treatment with surgery, radiation, or intensive cytostatic therapy. It is characterized by the hope of a cure. When metastasis is demonstrated, however, it may be difficult to decide between a new course of treatment, involving unpleasant side effects but also hope of a remission (curing), and palliative treatment (caring). Curing is generally regarded as active, and caring as passive. Health professionals often seem to become resigned when a cure seems unattainable. This is a completely mistaken attitude. Palliative treatment requires knowledge, diagnostic ability, and energetic action. Disseminated cancer is a multiorgan disease for which the clinician needs a broad knowledge of medicine to be able to help the patient. It represents a challenge to research and medical practice, and palliation is increasingly acknowledged to be an *active* form of treatment.

PART I

UNDERSTANDING PAIN

1

The Anatomy, Physiology, and Psychology of Pain

Over the last 20 years our knowledge of the pathways of pain in the central nervous system and of the physiological and psychological mechanisms of pain has made so much progress that it can almost be called a revolution. Before this, drugs and other therapy for relieving pain were used in a purely empirical way. Now, however, our new insight into the basic mechanisms of pain should lead to more rational and effective treatment.

Research in this field is difficult because of the subjective nature of pain. Objective findings are therefore difficult to establish. Animal models can be informative but have often been shown to be of little value in the human situation. Our knowledge is thus still full of gaps, in spite of all the progress that has been made. But there is a great deal of optimism in this field, and fresh knowledge is continually being discovered.

PERIPHERAL AND CENTRAL PATHWAYS OF PAIN

PERIPHERAL PATHWAYS

The body has peripheral nerves that are specially constructed to conduct pain impulses. There are probably many subgroups of pain fibers, but they are usually classified into two groups on the basis of their thickness, A-delta and C fibers. The C fibers are fine and unmyelinated and conduct impulses

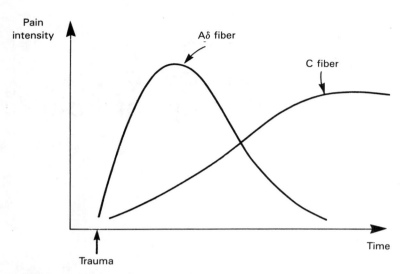

FIGURE 1. Activation of the A-delta and C primary afferent nociceptors.

relatively slowly (less than 2 m/s; see Fig. 1). They transmit the drilling, burning, deep, and lasting type of pain (protopathic pain). A-delta fibers are somewhat thicker and myelinated, they conduct impulses more rapidly (about 20 m/s), and they are responsible for transmitting stabbing, intense, superficial, short-lasting pain. Pressure, touch, vibration, and other sensations are conducted by the thicker, myelinated A-alpha and the somewhat finer A-delta fibers. This classification is mainly based on the study of pain receptors in the skin. The method of transmission of pain varies somewhat from organ to organ. For example, A-delta fibers from muscles can conduct the same type of pain as C fibers from skin.

The body is well supplied with nociceptors (pain receptors) in the skin, muscles, periosteum, peritendineum, parietal pleura and peritoneum, pericardium, capsules around the internal organs, and the tentorium/falx cerebri.

For a long time it was thought that the internal organs had no, or very few, nociceptors. Recently, however, the existence of nerves reacting to ischemia, inflammation, mechanical stretching, and other stimuli has been demonstrated in the heart, gastrointestinal tract, and other abdominal organs. The nerves that transmit nociceptive impulses also react to other sensory impulses; very strong impulses in these fibers seem to be perceived as pain. There is evidence, however, that some of these organs (at any rate the bile ducts) have specific pain fibers, that is, nerve endings that react only to painful stimuli. Pain from internal organs is conducted through fibers belonging to the autonomic (i.e., involuntary) nervous system, chiefly the sympathetic nervous system.

Mechanisms for the Occurrence of Nociceptive Pain in the Tissues

The nociceptors are activated by threatened or existing tissue destruction. Some A-delta fibers are activated by direct physical trauma (pressure), others by high or low temperature or chemical substances. The pain is conducted rapidly and strongly and with most types of stimuli will decrease fairly quickly (in the course of seconds to minutes), even if the painful stimulus continues. The function of this type of fiber thus seems to be to register changes in pain intensity, not to provide continuous information about pain, although some A-delta fibers can conduct pain impulses for a longer period.

C fibers are depolarized by the chemical substances formed during tissue injury, but they can also conduct nociceptive impulses caused by direct physical stimuli. The C fibers are activated more slowly than the A-delta fibers, but they conduct pain impulses for a long time after the injury and continue to transmit impulses actively as long as the stimulus lasts (see Fig. 1).

A number of substances produced by the body can cause pain when injected into tissue; examples are bradykinin, prostaglandins E_2 and I_2, histamine, serotonin, protons (low pH in the tissue), and potassium ions. There is a great deal we do not know about the physiological role of these substances in the pain process. It is possible that the different pain fibers react specifically to the different substances, but it is more likely that more than one of the substances has to be present at any time for nociceptive impulses to arise. Low doses of bradykinin do not normally give rise to pain, but they will do so if prostaglandin E_2 is also present. This is probably because the prostaglandin E_2 makes the pain fibers more sensitive to pain-provoking (algogenic) substances. Serotonin secreted from platelets has also been shown to potentiate the effect of bradykinin and acetylcholine.

All the above-mentioned algogenic substances are formed during tissue injury. Proteolytic enzymes in the injured area cleave the protein bradykininogen (plasma kininogen) that diffuses from the blood into the tissue fluid, forming bradykinin. Prostaglandin precursors are present in all cell membranes in the form of esterified fatty acids (phospholipids). If, for example, the tissue is injured, the phospholipids are cleaved by the enzyme phospholipase A_2, and arachidonic acid is formed (see Fig. 2). The enzyme cyclooxygenase can convert arachidonic acid to prostaglandins E_2 and F_2, prostacylin (prostaglandin I_2, or thromboxane, the type of prostaglandin being dependent on the cell type. Short-lived intermediary products like the prostaglandins G_2 and H_2 are also present in this reaction and probably also contribute to the arousal of pain. In some cells the arachidonic acid is also converted by the enzyme lipoxygenase to leukotrienes, which are potent mediators in the inflammatory process and may sensitize

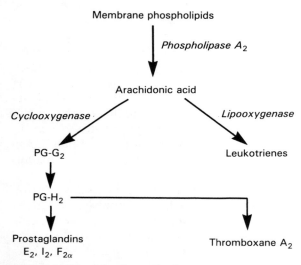

FIGURE 2. Prostaglandin synthesis.

nociceptors. Histamine from mast cells and potassium ions leaking out of injured cells can also depolarize nociceptors, and substance P released from primary afferent nerve fibers can sensitize them.

Nerve fibers that conduct pressure, tactile sensation, and so on require a weaker electrical stimulus than pain fibers in order to be activated. As we shall see later, this can be exploited clinically—for example, by the use of transcutaneous electrical nerve stimulation (see Fig. 3).

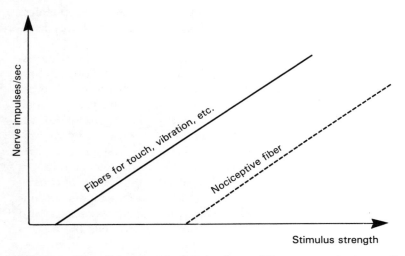

FIGURE 3. Effect of the strength of a stimulus on different types of primary afferent nerves.

Chronic Pain Can Lower the Pain Threshold

Many of the senses, like the sense of smell, adapt themselves to continuous stimulation. This means that the strength of the stimulus has to be increased to obtain the same response. The sense of pain in many cases shows the opposite tendency: chronic stimulation can lower the threshold, making the peripheral pain fibers more sensitive to new nociceptive impulses. The chemical mechanisms behind this are not clear.

Mechanisms for the Occurrence of Neuropathic Pain

Tissue injuries may involve injury to the nerve fibers, and within a short time the fibers will start to repair the injury (regeneration). The injured nerve puts out small sprouts to reinnervate the injured area of tissue. This is a very complicated process, however, and the sprouts can grow in the wrong direction, or form wrong connections or no connections at all, leading to the formation of a neuroma. A chronic active tissue injury like cancer or rheumatoid arthritis can create a state of almost continuous regeneration of nerve fibers and therefore of new sprouts. The sprouts may be:

1. Spontaneously active, that is, generate "pain" impulses without being influenced by algogenic (pain-producing) substances;
2. Hypersensitive to mechanical stimuli, so that a light touch or pressure on the tissue causes pain; or
3. Hypersensitive to norepinephrine or epinephrine from the sympathetic nervous system, so that pain is felt even with the normal concentrations of norepinephrine in the tissue.

If a nerve containing both motor and sensory fibers is injured, connections between different types of fibers may be formed during regeneration. These are known as ephapses. The result is that impulses from motor or sensory fibers are transmitted to pain fibers and produce pathological pain. A peripheral nerve injury will also cause changes in the central part of the nerve cell, in the dorsal root ganglion (see Fig. 4). These nerve cells can then be spontaneously activated and become hypersensitive to norepinephrine. Chronic changes in the neurons in the spinal cord may also occur (see below).

Neurotransmitters in Primary Afferent Nociceptive Nerve Fibers

The cell nuclei in the primary afferent sensory fibers are located in the dorsal root ganglion, where enzymes and transmitter substances are produced and from which they are transported both outward to the various tissues and inward to the spinal cord. Thus the primary afferent nerve fibers can release transmitter substances both peripherally to the tissues

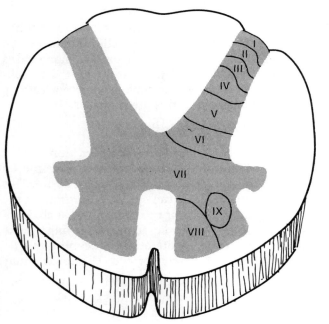

Lamina II = substantia gelatinosa

FIGURE 4. Laminas of the spinal cord.

and centrally in the spinal cord. Peptides such as substance P, vasoactive intestinal polypeptide (VIP), and cholecystokinin (CCK) have been demonstrated in C fibers (see also below). There is still a great deal we do not know about their functions, but substance P seems to be important in the transmission of nociceptive impulses in the dorsal horn of the spinal cord.

Substance P and other peptides are also secreted peripherally, in response to painful stimuli among other things, where they provoke strong vasodilation, inflammation, and sensitization of nociceptors. This phenomenon may be part of what is known as spreading secondary hyperalgesia, a condition where the nociceptors in adjacent areas are sensitized as well as those in the injured area. Thus the nervous system is involved in the genesis of inflammation and pain in response to injury.

SPINAL PATHWAYS

The impulses from sensory nerve fibers enter the dorsal root and are conducted into the dorsal horn of the spinal cord (gray matter; see Figs. 4 and 6). Impulses from C fibers, A-delta fibers, and visceral fibers are transmitted to different areas. The C fibers have synapses mainly in laminas I and II, the A-delta fibers mainly in laminas I and V, and the visceral fibers mainly in laminas I and V. The A-alpha and A-beta fibers, which conduct tactile sensation and other sensory stimuli, have synapses in laminas II and IV. The nociceptive fibers enter into synaptic relations in lamina I, and probably the outer part of lamina II, with cells that conduct the impulses to higher centers, mainly via the spinothalamic tract. There are no ascending fibers leading from lamina II (substantia gelatinosa), so impulses from this area have to be transmitted to the synapses in laminas I and V before they can be conducted upward in the spinal cord. The nociceptive afferent fibers send out collaterals to the motor neurons and nuclei in the autonomic nervous system in the spinal cord. These collaterals form part of the reflex arcs that lead to muscular tension and autonomic reactions in connection with pain.

The transmission of visceral pain is essentially different from that of other pain. There seem to be separate systems for the conduction of visceral pain impulses, but many of the primary afferent visceral nociceptive neurons have a synaptic relation with an ascending neuron that also transmits pain the skin and musculoskeletal tissues (see Fig. 5)—that is, a system where visceral and other somatic types of pain converge. The brain then sometimes interprets a visceral pain impulse as coming from the same place as a nonvisceral (somatic) pain impulse conducted by the same neuron. This is one probable mechanism behind referred pain and explains why, for example, the pain of a myocardial infarction can also be felt in the left arm.

Thus the brain receives impulses from several different levels in the dorsal horn and combines them to form a total picture. The farther the impulses travel in the dorsal horn, the more modified they become. The substantia gelatinosa (lamina II) is particularly important in this context. It consists of small neurons (interneurons) with short axons and dendrites that influence the transmission of pain.

ASCENDING PATHWAYS

At least five different systems have been found that carry information about pain from the spinal cord up to the brain. These are the spinothalamic tract, the reticulospinal tract, the spinomesencephalic tract, the

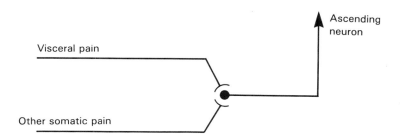

FIGURE 5. Probable mechanism of referred pain.

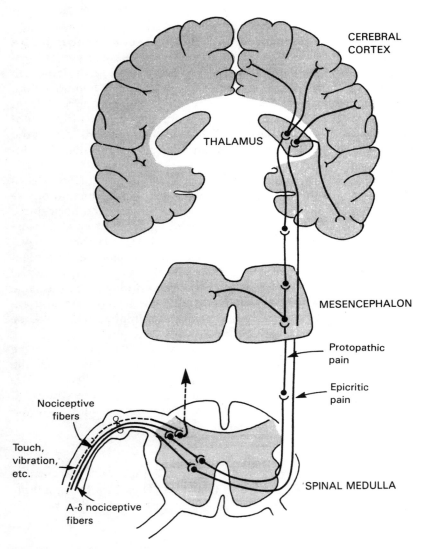

CEREBRAL
CORTEX

THALAMUS

MESENCEPHALON

Protopathic
pain

Epicritic
pain

Nociceptive
fibers

Touch,
vibration,
etc.

A-δ nociceptive
fibers

SPINAL MEDULLA

FIGURE 6. Nociceptive pathways in the central nervous system.

spinocervical tract, and a multisynaptic system in the spinal cord. These conduct pain impulses parallel to one another, but there is also contact between the systems. The spinothalamic tract is quantitatively the most important of the systems, and the others may be able to take over many of its functions if it is injured. After passing the synapse in a dorsal horn, most of the fibers cross the midline to the other side of the cord and ascend in the ventral or lateral spinothalamic tract (see Fig. 6). A certain number of the centrally conducting neurons, however, ascend ipsilaterally, without crossing over. A large proportion of the neurons that synapse with A-delta fibers are directly connected to the thalamus. Neurons that conduct C fiber impulses are connected directly and indirectly, via a polysynaptic system, to the reticular substance, autonomic brain stem nuclei, and hypothalamus. This is why people are kept awake by pain and why it can be associated with autonomic disturbances like nausea, raised blood pressure, cold sweating, and so on.

THALAMOCORTICAL PATHWAYS

The pain impulses from the thalamus are thought to be transmitted in five main directions.

1. The *primary sensory area*, which corresponds to the postcentral gyrus, lies just behind the central sulcus. The function of the impulses to this area is mainly to localize the pain and distinguish the types of pain (see Fig. 7).
2. The *secondary sensory area* (area of association) lies farther back in the parietal lobe. It probably helps to interpret the character and significance of a pain.

The various components of a pain—the origin, physical quality (burning, pricking, etc.), intensity, and so on—are distinguished and iden-

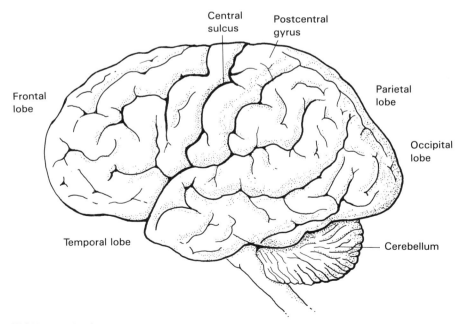

FIGURE 7. Surface anatomy of the brain.

tified in these two areas. Thus these parts of the brain register the bare facts about the pain.

3. The *limbic system* (the "emotional brain") is a common term for a number of different-sized groups of nuclei, including the amygdaloid body, the nuclei of the septum, the hippocampus, the gyrus cinguli, and the preoptic region of the hypothalamus. These areas interpret the emotional, or affective, component of the pain. This is where pain "really hurts." A person's emotions, such as anxiety or depression, will affect the interpretation of the pain, and the pain, in its turn, will affect the emotions. Thus the emotional implications of the pain help determine its severity or painfulness, and there is a close interaction between the emotional component of a pain and other emotions. Large numbers of efferent fibers connect the limbic system with other areas of the brain, the brain stem, and the spinal medulla, and, as we shall see, it influence the transmission of pain.
4. An important region of the memory is situated in the *temporal lobe*. Protracted pain and repeated pain are usually the kinds that are most indelibly stored, and the remembrance of pain makes fresh pain more easily felt. If a patient can be kept free of pain over a certain period, the memory of pain becomes blurred, and new pain is less easily initiated.
5. The *frontal cortex* is also deeply involved in the perception and processing of the intensity and significance of a pain. Cognitive processes can therefore affect the perception of pain. This can be exploited therapeutically.

ENDOGENOUS PAIN-INHIBITING MECHANISMS

The knowledge that the body has mechanisms for moderating pain is not new. An athlete who is injured during a game often does not notice the pain until afterward. Two people who have broken the same bone in their bodies can experience the pain quite differently. A patient with a compression fracture in a vertebral body caused by an injury usually finds it easier to bear the pain than a patient with a compression fracture caused by metastasizing cancer. Why? Until about 20 years ago the reasons for these differences were very unclear, but since then our knowledge of the underlying mechanisms has increased at an exponential rate.

At the beginning of the 1970s morphine was shown to bind specific receptors in the nervous tissue. Why should the human brain contain a receptor for a plant alkaloid like morphine? Could it be that the real function of these receptors was to bind the body's own morphinelike substances? Later, two pentapeptides with a high affinity to these receptors were located. They were termed enkephalins, from the Greek *enkephalos*, meaning "the brain." Thus it was discovered that nervous tissue synthesizes specific pain-inhibiting substances. During the last 10 years there has been an explosive development in research in this area, and three families of substances have been found that bind to opioid receptors ("morphine receptors") and have an analgesic effect: the beta-endorphin family, the enkephalin family, and the dynorphin family. The common name for all of these substances is *endorphins* or *endogenous opioid peptides*. They are peptides with 5 to 31 amino acids. The five N-terminal amino acids tyrosine-glycine-glycine-phenylalanine-leucine/methionine are common to all the peptides and are necessary for the opioid receptor affinity.

PEPTIDE NEURONS

Along with the endorphins, a number of other peptides were found that function as transmitters in the nervous system. It is important to distinguish between this group of substances and other transmitters. Peptides are molecules that consist of amino acids joined together in rows. Those with few amino acids are known as oligopeptides, and those with a larger number are known as polypeptides or proteins.

There are clear-cut differences between the "classical" transmitter substances, such as acetylcholine and serotonin, and neuropeptides. Neurons that release classical transmitters produce enzymes in the body of the cell, which are transported through the axons to the nerve terminal. There they synthesize the transmitter substance, which is then stored in small vesicles. When the nerve terminal receives impulses, the transmitters are liberated into the synaptic cleft and provoke a rapid response in the next cell in the form of an action potential. Shortly afterward most of the transmitter substance is either taken up again by the presynaptic terminal and re-stored in the vesicles, or it is cleaved by enzymes in the synaptic cleft. The transmitters are rapidly resynthesized, ready for use (see Fig. 8).

Peptide neurons synthesize propeptides in the form of proteins with molecular weights of 10,000 to 40,000 and store them in vesicles close to the nucleus. The vesicles are transported in the axon to the nerve terminal. This takes from 30 minutes to 24 hours. During the transport, enzymes cleave the propeptides, leading to the formation of active peptides, which are stored in presynaptic vesicles. The release of peptides into the synaptic cleft may provoke an action potential in the postsynaptic neuron, but peptides often function more as neuromodulators or neurohormones than purely as neurotransmitters. That is, they act on neurons and alter them qualitatively, for example, by making them less sensitive to excitation by classical transmitters. Many of the peptides are not broken down to any great extent in the synaptic cleft and can therefore diffuse over a broad area, influencing a large number of cells and having a long-lasting effect. Peptides are not usually taken up again in the presynaptic terminal.

Recent research has shown that classical transmitters and neuropeptides can be produced in the same neuron. The various transmitters can

Classical transmitter neuron | Peptide neuron

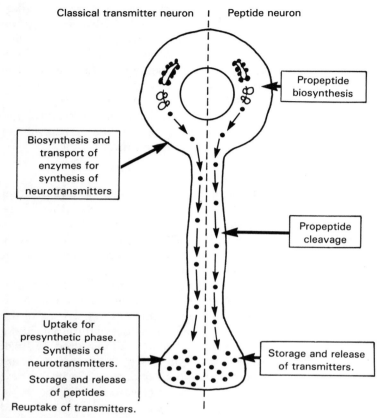

Propeptide
biosynthesis

Biosynthesis and
transport of
enzymes for
synthesis of
neurotransmitters

Propeptide
cleavage

Uptake for
presynthetic phase.
Synthesis of
neurotransmitters.

Storage and release
of peptides

Reuptake of transmitters.

Storage and release
of transmitters.

FIGURE 8. Diagram of the properties of classical neurotransmitter neurons and peptide neurons. (Adapted from T. Hökfelt et al., Nature, 284:515–521, 1980.)

also act on different effector cells or modify each other's effect on the same effector cell. Classical transmitters and peptides can also be released at different times and in response to different stimuli. We have thus become aware that the central nervous system functions in a much more complicated and differentiated way than was thought even a few years ago.

BIOSYNTHESIS AND OCCURRENCE OF ENDOGENOUS OPIOID PEPTIDES

Endogenous opioid peptides are classified in families according to the protein, or propeptide, from which they are cleaved. See Fig. 9 and Table 1.

The distribution of endogenous opioid peptides differs widely. Nerve cells containing beta-endorphins are situated in the hypothalamus. They have long axons extending into the brain stem and the limbic system. The pituitary gland also contains large amounts of endorphins, which are released into the blood and may also be carried to the brain by the portal circulation, but this has not been definitely demonstrated. The endorphins secreted by the pituitary gland are acetylated and in this form have no analgesic effect. They have to be deacetylated in order to inhibit pain, and whether this occurs in the body is not known.

Enkephalin-producing neurons have been found in laminas I, II, and IV in the dorsal horn, in the brain stem, near the aqueduct and the third ventricle in the mesencephalon and the diencephalon, and in several areas of the limbic system. Altogether, enkephalin-producing neurons have been found in over 20 cell groups in the central nervous system, and most of them consist of small interneurons. Neurons containing dynorphin are usually also interneurons and are found in much the same areas as the enkephalins. Outside the central nervous system these peptides have

Pro-opiomelanocortin

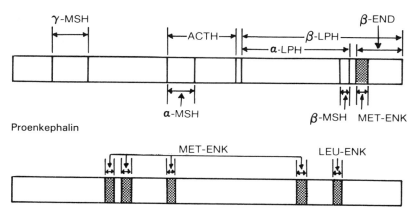

Proenkephalin

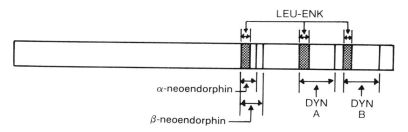

Prodynorphin

FIGURE 9. The propeptides of various endogenous opioid peptides. ENK = enkephalin, DYN = dynorphin, END = endorphin, MSH = melanocyte-stimulating hormone, ACTH = adrenocorticotropic hormone, LPH = lipotropin.

TABLE 1. Classification of Endogenous Opioid Peptides

Propeptide	Most important peptides
Pro-opiomelanocortin	Beta-endorphin
	Melanocyte-stimulating hormone (MSH)
	Adrenocorticotropic hormone (ACTH)
Proenkephalin A	Enkephalins
Prodynorphin	Dynorphin
	Alpha-neoenkephalin

been found in the medulla of the adrenal gland and in the gastrointestinal and urogenital tracts.

SPINAL GATE CONTROL

Briefly, this mechanism is based on the fact that activation of sensory afferent fibers (for example, those for touch and vibration) can relieve pain. The site of inhibition of the pain impulse is the dorsal horn of the spinal cord. The effect is rapid and ceases soon after removal of the mechanical stimulus. Stimulation must take place in the area where the pain originates, although contralateral stimulation also has some effect. Methods that seem to activate this mechanism are massage, hot and cold packs, and high-frequency transcutaneous electrical nerve stimulation (TENS).

The sites of inhibition of the pain are lamina I (the marginal zone) and lamina II (substantia gelatinosa) in the dorsal horn of the spinal cord. The best effect is obtained with protopathic (deep-seated, aching) pain in C fibers and sometimes in neuropathic pain. The effect on epicritic (intense, rapid, stabbing) pain in the A-delta fibers is less good.

The nociceptive afferents that enter the dorsal horn have synapses in lamina I and the outer part of the substantia gelatinosa. Other afferent sensory fibers have synapses in the inner part of the substantia gelatinosa. The primary afferent sensory nociceptive fibers have opioid receptors. The neurotransmitter in many of these neurons is probably substance P, a peptide with 11 amino acids. A large number of interneurons containing enkephalin, dynorphin, and other inhibitory neurotransmitters like gamma-aminobutyric acid (GABA) have been shown to be present in laminas I and II, but it is not clear how the impulses in the sensory fibers inhibit the pain impulses, although there are a number of theories about it.

An early theory was that thick sensory fibers stimulate enkephalin-secreting interneurons that inhibit nociceptive impulses presynaptically (see Fig. 10a). Evidence for this theory is that the primary nociceptive neuron has presynaptic opioid receptors and that endogenous opioids are very probably involved in the gate control. However, enkephalin neurons have not been shown to have synaptic connections with primary afferents, only with the centrally conducting neuron. In spite of this, it is possible that presynaptic inhibition does take place, caused by, for example, dynorphin. Enkephalins can probably diffuse into the tissue and cause presynaptic inhibition even without direct synapses.

There are thus morphological reasons for maintaining that inhibition of pain impulses occurs postsynaptically. It may be due to endogenous opioids (enkephalin and dynorphin) or other inhibitory substances like GABA.

Recent findings indicate, however, that the situation is more complicated. The primary afferent C fibers have no direct synaptic connections with the ascending second-order neurons in the spinothalamic tract. The impulse is relayed through one or more excitatory interneurons, which in turn are influenced by both excitatory and inhibitory interneurons (see

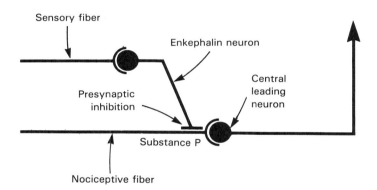

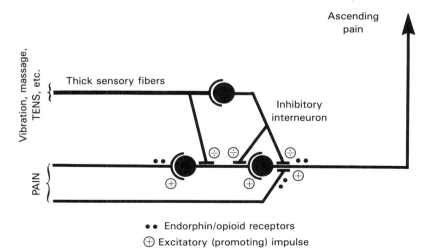

•• Endorphin/opioid receptors
⊕ Excitatory (promoting) impulse
⊖ Inhibitory impulse

FIGURE 10. (a) Early model of spinal gate control. (b) More recent model of spinal gate control.

Fig. 10b). The impulses transmitted from here are the summation of all these modifying factors. In other words, in their progress through the dorsal horn nociceptive impulses are influenced by a number of neurons and transmitter substances. Figure 10b shows some of the connections between the cells in the dorsal horn and those involved in the transmission of pain. Primary nociceptive neurons send most of their impulses through excitatory interneurons, and here we do not know which transmitters are liberated. Some of the pain impulses are relayed directly to second-order ascending neurons and some to inhibitory interneurons, so that in fact pain can inhibit pain. Thick sensory fibers have synaptic connections with inhibitory interneurons, which can weaken the impulses in the excitatory interneuron or in the ascending pain fiber. The sensory fibers also have direct synaptic connections with excitatory interneurons and may be able to inhibit them. The figure also shows neurons with opioid receptors that bind morphine, enkephalin, and dynorphin.

There is evidence for a thalamic gate control analogous to the spinal one, but much less is known about this.

DESCENDING SYSTEMS
FOR THE MODULATION OF PAIN

Electrical stimulation of the brain cells in animals around the third ventricle and along the cerebral aqueduct at the fourth ventricle and of centrally situated nuclei in the brain stem (raphe nuclei) has been found to be strongly analgesic. These areas are known as the periventricular gray matter (PVG), the periaqueductal gray matter (PAG), and the nucleus raphe magnus (NRM). Severe chronic pain can be relieved to some extent in humans by the stimulation of corresponding areas, but without such good results as in the animal studies. This is probably because of the more complicated anatomy and physiology of the human body; it is also very difficult to position the electrodes correctly in humans.

The presence of considerable numbers of opioid receptors has been demonstrated in the PAG, and microinjection of morphine into the PAG, NRM, and neighboring areas in the medulla oblongata has resulted in the same degree of analgesia as with electrical stimulation. If the descending pathways from this area are severed, the analgesic effect ceases. This means that the inhibition of pain does not take place in the mesencephalon and the medulla oblongata, but through the descending pathways that cause the dorsal horn to inhibit impulses at that level.

Thus, the most important centers of endogenous pain inhibition are the PAG in the mesencephalon, the rostral ventral medulla (RVM), including the NRM, and the dorsal horn of the spinal cord. These three areas will therefore be described in more detail below. (See Fig. 11.)

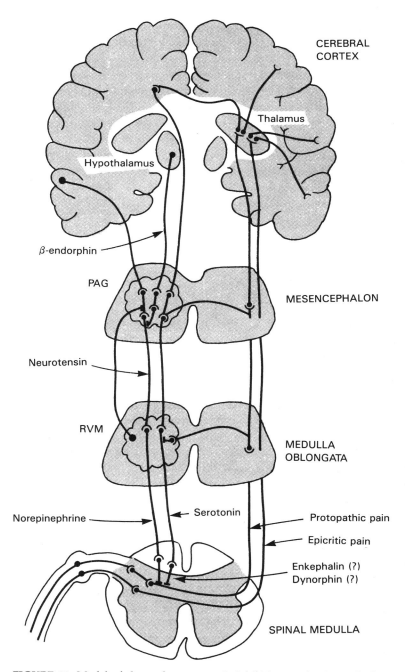

FIGURE 11. Model of the endogenous pain-inhibiting mechanisms. PAG = periaqueductal gray substance, RVM = rostral ventral medulla.

The Periaqueductal Gray Matter

Both electrical stimulation and microinjection of opiates into the PAG have a strong analgesic effect. The area contains many opioid receptors and many interneurons secreting enkephalin and dynorphin. Most of the incoming stimuli to the PAG are borne by long beta-endorphin-containing neurons that originate in the hypothalamus. This pathway is probably an important one in endogenous pain inhibition. The PAG also has afferent connections with the cerebral cortex and the limbic system (the insula and the amygdala), which may indicate that cognitive and emotional factors directly influence the pain-inhibiting process. The PAG is also connected by collaterals from the spinothalamic tract (the "pain pathway"). Input to the PAG is also provided by the locus ceruleus, a group of cells in the pons that produce norepinephrine as a neurotransmitter. This pathway appears to inhibit the analgesic effect of the PAG.

The Rostral Ventral Medulla Including the Nucleus Raphe Magnus

Descending pathways extend from the PAG to the RVM, probably with the peptide neorotensin as a major neurotransmitter. The RVM also receives information from the hypothalamus and from nociceptive impulses in the spinothalamic tract. This can act as a negative feedback mechanism, where pain inhibits pain. The region contains many interneurons liberating enkephalin, dynorphin, and other transmitters.

The Descending Pathways to the Dorsal Horn

Descending pathways lead from the NRM through the dorsolateral tract to the dorsal horn of the spinal cord. Serotonin (5-HT) and norepinephrine have been shown to be quantitatively the most important transmitters in these pathways. In addition, the dorsal horn receives pain-inhibiting impulses from other nuclei in the medulla oblongata, the nucleus paragigantocellularis, and the noradrenergic medullary group of cells. The events that take place when the descending pathways enter the dorsal horn resemble those described under Spinal Gate Control above. This means that the inhibitory interneurons liberate enkephalin, dynorphin, and other transmitters to inhibit the pain impulses in the ascending pain neuron (postsynaptically), but probably presynaptic inhibition also occurs, even though no direct enkephalin or dynorphin synapses have been demonstrated here. Direct postsynaptic inhibition also occurs in serotonergic descending neurons.

WHICH PHYSIOLOGICAL FACTORS INHIBIT PAIN?

There is no doubt that stimulation, whether electrical or by opioid administration, of the systems described above has a strongly analgesic effect.

We know less, however, about how these systems function physiologically. There is good evidence that pain activates the pain-inhibiting systems: many people have described how the pain in their back was relieved by toothache! Popular medicine has long made use of this principle and has used techniques like cupping, mustard plasters, and certain types of painful stimuli to relieve chronic pain. In many animal experiments painful stimuli applied to one area of the body have been shown to relieve pain at another. These experiments indicate that there are several different pain-inhibiting systems. Some act rapidly, within minutes or seconds. Others usually require 15–30 minutes of pain stimulation before they become effective. There are many other factors, however, that influence the efficiency of pain relief, such as psychological factors, the patient's ability to control the pain, the type and intensity of the pain, and the duration of the pain. (See Fig. 12.)

Nonpainful stimuli can also activate the endogenous pain-inhibiting mechanisms. Touch, massage, and muscular activity have been shown to bring relief, and so have transcutaneous electrical nerve stimulation and acupuncture. As I shall discuss later, psychological factors have an enormous influence on the perception of pain. Stress can strongly activate pain-inhibiting mechanisms and produce analgesia—when we are very frightened we do not feel pain. In animal experiments this stress-induced analgesia has been shown to be reversed to some extent by the morphine receptor antagonist naloxone.

There is no definite correlation between the level of endorphin in the blood and pain relief, even though several studies have appeared to indicate this. The endorphin in the blood comes mainly from the pituitary gland, and thus has to pass through the blood-brain barrier before it can act as a painreliever. Only small amounts do pass through, and these are acetylated and thus not active as an analgesic. As mentioned above, the endorphin is secreted together with ACTH, which may aggravate pain. It is interesting that in some experiments stress-induced analgesia has been attenuated after adrenalectomy. Adrenal medullary chromaffin cells synthe-

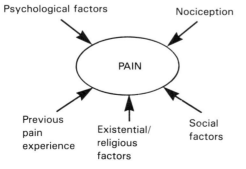

FIGURE 12. Factors that influence the experience of pain.

size large amounts of enkephalins, which are released during stress and may be distributed to the central nervous system and produce analgesia.

There does seem to be a connection, however, between the concentration of endogenous opioid peptides in the cerebrospinal fluid and the degree of pain relief. In a study in which endogenous opioid peptides in the cerebrospinal fluid were quantitated, it was found that the patients with the highest concentrations were least in need of postoperative analgesics. Patients with chronic somatic pain may have decreased concentrations of endogenous opioid peptides in cerebrospinal fluid. Patients with so-called chronic psychogenic pain have normal or increased levels. Healthy people differ in the amounts of endogenous opioid peptides found in the cerebrospinal fluid, and this may explain why the reaction to and tolerance of pain vary so much from person to person.

Although most research has been concerned with pain-*inhibiting* mechanisms, it has also been discovered that the body has important pain-*provoking* mechanisms, which facilitate the transmission of pain impulses and increase pain. The intensity of pain may therefore depend on the balance between these systems.

PHARMACOLOGICAL MANIPULATION OF ENDOGENOUS PAIN INHIBITION

The endogenous pain-inhibiting mechanisms described above involve neurons that are serotonergic, dopaminergic, noradrenergic, or cholinergic as well as neurons with endogenous opioid peptides and other peptides as neurotransmitters. A number of studies have been done on animal models to see what effect these transmitters have on pain relief.

Serotonin

Serotonin antagonists usually reduce the analgesia produced by morphine or by electrical stimulation of certain areas of the central nervous system, like the PAG, RVM, and NRM. On the other hand, an increase in serotonin concentration may potentiate analgesia. This is especially interesting since depression is thought to be accompanied by decreased concentrations of serotonin in the nerve terminals. This may help to explain why depressed patients sometimes have a reduced tolerance to pain and why antidepressants that act on serotonin metabolism can increase pain tolerance. The serotonin concentration is also increased by acupuncture. Tricyclic antidepressants can enhance the effects of acupuncture and transcutaneous electrical nerve stimulation.

Acetylcholine

Centrally acting cholinergics have been shown in some experiments to have an independent analgesic effect that is not related to the endogenous opioid peptide system, but relatively little is known about this. Centrally acting anticholinergics have been shown to decrease analgesia in animal experiments, and their use in humans has been accompanied by an increase in pain.

Dopamine

Some animal experiments have shown that an increased dopamine concentration produces increased analgesia, while others have shown the opposite. In experiments with humans, apomorphine (a dopamine receptor agonist) reduces the analgesia obtained with acupuncture, while droperidol (a dopamine receptor antagonist) increases analgesia. There is some evidence that certain neuroleptics (dopamine receptor antagonists) increase morphine-induced analgesia, although this has not been shown to have any clinical importance. This applies to low-dose neuroleptics and methotrimeprazine. This effect has not been demonstrated with any certainty for other high-dose neuroleptics.

Norepinephrine

The descending norepinephrine pathways are very important for the suppression of pain in the dorsal horn, and intraspinal administration of norepinephrine agonists increases analgesia. The presence of norepinephrine, in the mesencephalon, however, lessens analgesia. The effect on pain of drugs with an affinity for noradrenergic receptors cannot be predicted.

THE PLACEBO EFFECT

Placebos can give temporary relief from pain in about 30–50% of patients. A number of studies have shown that naloxone (an endorphin receptor antagonist) can counteract the effect of a placebo. This indicates that in some people the placebo effect may be partly due to the person's activation of the endogenous opioid peptide system in the brain by psychological mechanisms. Nonendorphinergic pain-inhibiting mechanisms can also be activated by psychological factors. We thus know a little about the structural and biochemical mechanisms behind the placebo effect, and we should try to make use of this knowledge to give patients the greatest confidence in our methods of treating pain.

AN INTRODUCTION TO PAIN PSYCHOLOGY

The nature of pain is difficult to define because it is a personal and subjective experience. It consists of two components, the sensory/discriminating and the emotional/cognitive (see p. 00). The emphasis on the relative importance of the two components has varied over the years, and modern medicine has tended to overemphasize the first, by regarding pain as a simple stimulus-response phenomenon, the emotional component being seen as a *reaction* to the physical stimulus of pain. This view has led to widespread experimental research into pain, but is has also led to the emotional aspects being considered "irrelevant." Recent research, however, has clearly shown that the perception of pain is the *total sum* of the somatic pain stimuli, the implications of the pain, and the thoughts and feelings of the patient. This means that social and existential factors also strongly influence the experience of pain. Thus, the psychological component is just as important as the somatic/sensory component. One consequence of this is the realization that somatic pain stimuli affect a patient's psychological functioning. Another is that the emotional and cognitive processing of pain can be utilized therapeutically. Methods like hypnosis, biofeedback, various forms of suggestion, imagery, distraction, and so on have repeatedly been shown to increase the patient's ability to cope with the pain.

DIFFERENCES BETWEEN ACUTE AND CHRONIC PAIN

There are very clear-cut physiological and psychological differences between acute and chronic pain. Acute pain usually arises in connection with an injury or an acute disease. Anxiety is often the dominating emotional component in the experience of acute pain, yet such pain is generally felt to be much less serious than chronic pain. This is because it is meaningful; the sense of pain causes us to notice tissue injury and to set in motion the necessary measures for counteracting the injury or disease. Our sense of pain enables us to avoid injury and is a constant reminder to us to avoid movement in injured parts of the body so as to facilitate the healing process. Pain thus enables us to remain healthy, as can be seen from the fact that people born without a sense of pain have significantly shorter life expectancies. Because acute pain is meaningful and because it is expected to cease in response to treatment, it is far easier to bear than chronic pain.

Chronic pain appears meaningless because it no longer functions as a reminder of a disease that can be treated and cured. It makes no sense for an otherwise healthy person to suffer chronic pain for the rest of his or her life from postherpetic or trigeminal neuralgia. Pain in such situations serves no purpose; on the contrary, it merely debilitates the sufferer. It also seems meaningless for a cancer patient to suffer constant pains in the back that only serve as a reminder that the cancer has spread to the spinal column. Living with chronic pain causes the patient to sleep badly, eat too little and lose weight, become depressed, and generally become too worn down to fight against the disease. Pain can thus shorten the patient's life. Chronic pain can dominate people's thoughts to the exclusion of everything else, absorbing all their concentration and draining all their strength. This has important psychological consequences, and patients with chronic pain often have symptoms that resemble those of depression. They have difficulty in sleeping and are irritable and lacking in energy. They feel depressed and can see no solution to their problems. Sometimes chronic pain seems to change the whole personality. Cheerful, extroverted people can become depressed, introverted, and bitter within weeks or even days. It is therefore extremely important for the patient, the patient's family, and the medical staff that the pain is taken seriously and given proper treatment.

Acute pain gives rise to a number of reactions in the autonomic sympathetic nervous system:

- Changes, generally an increase, in the blood pressure and pulse rate.
- Increased respiratory frequency.
- Pupillary dilatation.
- Cold sweating.
- Peripheral vasoconstriction with pale skin.
- Reduced motility in the gastrointestinal tract.

The secretion of the stress hormones norepinephrine and cortisol is also greatly increased. If the pain stimuli last for a long time these reactions begin to diminish, and patients with chronic pain usually have very insignificant autonomic reactions, so that the fact that they are suffering is not always obvious. There are usually no increased levels of stress hormones.

2

Assessment of Pain

In any field of clinical medicine it is extremely important to make sure that the diagnosis is correct as far as possible before beginning treatment. In the case of pain, however, this principle is often neglected. Many physicians seem satisfied to note that "the patient complains of pain" and proceed to prescribe a standard dose of an analgesic. If this has no effect they try a standard dose of a similar preparation, usually with the same result.

When a patient complains of pain, it is essential to try to discover the kind of pain the patient is suffering from and what is causing it. The method of treatment can then be varied according to the type of pain to be dealt with. Improvement in the treatment of pain depends on the pain being correctly diagnosed.

This chapter deals with the assessment of pain. The various treatments available are listed where appropriate and will be described in detail in Chapter 10.

TYPES OF PAIN

Pain can be divided into the following types: (1) pain caused by tissue injury (nociceptive, "normal," physiological pain), (2) pain caused by nerve injury or disease of the central nervous system (neuropathic pain, neuralgia), (3) referred pain, and (4) pain caused by psychological factors.

NOCICEPTIVE ("NORMAL," PHYSIOLOGICAL PAIN)

This type of pain is caused by tissue injury that stimulates the nociceptors directly or acts via pain-producing (algogenic) agents (bradykinin, prostaglandins, etc.). Terms commonly used to describe it are nociception, normal pain, and physiological pain.

Nociceptive pain originates from three structures: the skin, the musculoskeletal system (deep-seated somatic pain), and the internal organs (visceral pain). The skin is densely innervated by nociceptors to ensure a rapid withdrawal reflex to avoid extensive injury. The musculoskeletal system is also innervated by A-delta and C primary afferent fibers, but less densely than the skin. This implies a less precise location of the pain. The nociceptors respond to tissue injury, inflammation, and ischemia. Nociceptive impulses from deep-seated somatic structures often give rise to referred pain. Visceral pain stimuli are transmitted through the autonomic system, mainly through the sympathetic nervous system, but they may also be relayed through somatic pain fibers if the disease causing the pain affects the body wall. Visceral pain is usually diffuse, poorly localized, and felt over a large area. It is generally referred to sites other than the affected organ. Acute pain of visceral origin is often accompanied by autonomic reactions such as an increase in heart rate and blood pressure, sweating, and pale skin. Motor reflexes with increased tension in abdominal muscles may also be evident. Visceral pain is often caused by distension of hollow viscera or organ capsules, or by inflammation and ischemia. On the other hand, cutting, heat, pinching, and even the presence of large tumors may not elicit pain.

Nociceptive pain can be described as follows:

Epicritic pain. Rapid, superficial stabbing pain conducted (at any rate from the skin) through the thick myelinated A-delta fibers. This term covers the following kinds of clinical pain: pain from stings and cuts, movement-related pain associated with fractures and soft tissue injuries, and colic. The response to ordinary analgesics varies.

Protopathic pain. This is slow, deep-seated, throbbing pain, difficult to locate, which is conducted through fine, unmyelinated C fibers. This kind of pain occurs in connection with tissue injury caused by tumors, inflammation (e.g., from infection, rheumatism), ischemia (infarction), mechanical tissue injury, and so forth. The response to analgesics is usually good.

NEUROPATHIC PAIN (NEUROGENIC PAIN, NEURALGIA)

Neuropathic pain is caused by injury to the nerve structures in the peripheral and/or the central nervous system. The pain arises because the injured nerve structures react abnormally to stimuli that usually give rise to little or no pain, or the nerve fibers may be spontaneously activated and transmit pain without any exogenous stimulus. Injured nerves may be (1) hypersensitive to norepinephrine, so that normal or only slightly increased activity in the sympathetic nervous system can give rise to pain, or (2) hypersensitive to touch, so that a slight pressure on the nerves can give rise to considerable pain.

A number of terms are used to describe the various kinds of neuropathic pain. The definitions are adapted from *Pain*, Supplement 3, 1986.

Neuralgia: "nerve pains" in the area supplied by the nerve(s).

Hyperalgesia: an increased response to a stimulus that is normally painful.

Hyperpathia: increased reaction to a repetitive stimulus as well as a higher threshold.

Dysesthesia: an unpleasant abnormal sensation, whether spontaneous or provoked. In the assessment of pain the term is often used to describe pricking, burning pains, usually in superficial structures (skin).

Allodynia: pain triggered by stimuli that normally do not cause pain, such as a light touch on the skin.

Causalgia: continuous, burning pain, allodynia and hyperpathia, following injury to nerve(s), combined with vasomotor disturbances (vasoconstriction or vasodilation) and trophic changes such as skin atrophy, muscular atrophy, and sometimes skeletal decalcification.

Deafferentation pain: pain caused by complete or incomplete nerve lesions.

Central pain: pain caused by an injury to the central nervous system, such as by a tumor or infarction ("stroke"). Such pain is often due to an injury in the brain stem (medulla oblongata, pons, mesencephalon), the diencephalon (thalamus, capsula interna), or the cortex cerebri. The pain is thus usually spread over a large area, such as the whole of one side of the body.

Stabbing, lancinating pain: paroxysmal, radiating pain, usually in connection with neuralgia.

Neuropathic pain occurs after nerve injuries caused by surgery, radiotherapy, cytostatic drugs (*Vinca* alkaloids, cisplatin), and tumor infiltration and may also be caused by chronic tissue injury giving rise to secondary damage to nerves (chronic inflammation, rheumatism).

REFERRED PAIN

This term describes pain that arises in deep-seated structures or organs and that the patient experiences in another part of the body, usually the skin or some other superficial structure. One reason for this is that visceral and deep somatic nociceptive impulses are conveyed to the same ascending neurons in the spinal cord as pain from, for example, the skin. The brain therefore interprets the pain as coming from the superficial structure as well (see p. 9). Clinical examples of this phenomenon are the pain from a myocardial infarction perceived in the left arm and abdominal pain involving irritation of the diaphragm that gives rise to pain in the shoulder on the same side. Pain in the musculoskeletal system is often referred to areas some distance from the pathological process. Referred pain makes diagnosis difficult, particularly since the site of referred pain is often tender when palpated, which can mislead both the physician and the patient into believing that this site is the seat of the disease process.

PAIN CAUSED BY PSYCHOLOGICAL FACTORS

In psychotic patients imaginary pain may be the only symptom, but usually it occurs together with other hallucinations, as part of the disease. In neurotic patients pain may originate from muscular tension or psychosomatic disease, or it may be purely a conversion phenomenon—that is, without any somatic basis. Pain in a conversion disorder or psychogenic pain disorder closely resembles that in somatic disease but is often described in vague terms and does not correspond to anatomical structures. On the other hand, somatic pain may follow an atypical path: neuropathic pain from partial nerve lesions often does not conform to dermatomes, and pain in the musculoskeletal system can be referred to the most surprising anatomical sites (radiating along myotomes or sclerotomes). Somatic pain can therefore easily be mistaken in many cases for a conversion disorder or psychogenic pain disorder. For the diagnosis "psychogenic pain" to be valid, a lack of somatic basis for the pain must be accompanied by psychopathology. Many patients receive an unfounded psychiatric diagnosis because of a lack of diagnostic expertise. It is important to realize that psychogenic pain can be as distressing to the patient as somatic pain. The physician must therefore take these patients' symptoms seriously and not dismiss them as being merely imagination. What a patient experiences as pain *is* pain. It is the physician's task to discover the components of the pain and to treat them correctly.

CLINICAL CLASSIFICATION OF PAIN

There is considerable disagreement about the classification of pain, but I have found that the following categories are clinically useful:

A1. Acute
  2. Chronic
B1. Nociceptive
  2. Neuropathic
  3. Psychogenic

A clinical pain condition is a combination of A and B. Labor pains are acute and nociceptive, while the pain associated with a postherpetic neuralgia is chronic an neuropathic. A cancer patient with metastasis to the spine, compression fractures, and pressure on the nerves will be suffering from chronic, nociceptive, neuropathic pain. In some cases it may be useful to subdivide pain into acute, subacute, and chronic and acute recurring and chronic recurring conditions.

PAIN HISTORY

The most important points to clarify are the site of the pain; the type of pain; the intensity of the pain; factors that aggravate or alleviate the pain; variations in the pain over time; the patient's response to previous treatment of the pain; and the effect of emotional, social, and existential (spiritual) factors on the patient's experience of the pain.

SITE OF THE PAIN

The site of the pain should be pinpointed as accurately as possible so that its origin can be correctly determined. A diagram of the body is useful here for charting the areas and types of pain (see Figs. 13 and 14). This is a simple and effective diagnostic aid, which also helps the physician to plot the course of the pain, especially in cases where more than one physician is involved in the treatment. It facilitates communication between colleagues. Some prefer the physician to fill in the diagram, but the best and most effective method is for the patient to fill it in. The depth of the pain should also be registered—that is, whether the patient feels the pain in a superficial structure like the skin or in deep-seated tissue. The patient should also be asked whether the pain is radiating and, if so, where.

TYPE OF PAIN

The health professional should try to distinguish between nociceptive, neuropathic, referred, and psychogenic pain. The response to analgesics varies considerably with the type of pain. Deep, aching somatic pain, pain in bones, and so on usually respond well to ordinary analgesics, but the effect of the latter on the various forms of neuropathic pain is very limited.

Movement-related pain also tends to respond poorly to classical analgesics.

INTENSITY OF THE PAIN

It is difficult, but important, to quantitate pain. Since pain is a subjective experience made up of somatic signals, emotions, motivation, cognition, and much else, it is obviously hard to quanitate its intensity. The following scale, for example, is used by many researchers, who ask the patient to fill it in:

- No pain.
- Slight pain.
- Moderate pain.
- Severe pain.

(a) Name:
 Date of birth:
 Indicate the site(s)
 of pain on the drawing.
 Describe the pain, using
 one or more of the letters
 below at each site.
 A: stabbing pain
 B: burning pain
 C: deep-seated, aching pain
 D: sharp prickling pain
 E: pinching, constricting pain

(b) Indicate the severity
 of the pain by putting
 a cross on the line below:

No_____Unbearable
pain   pain

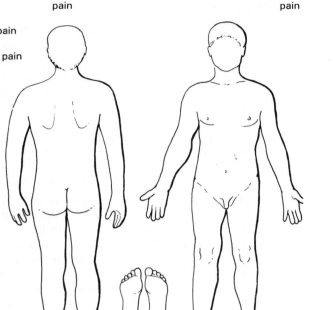

FIGURE 13. Body chart for indicating areas and types of pain. (b) Visual analog scale.

In recent years the visual analog scale (VAS), a simple, practical, and reproducible method for measuring pain, has been widely used. The patient makes a cross on a 100-mm-long straight line, running from painlessness on the left to unbearable pain on the right. The cross indicates the patient's assessment of the pain in relation to these two poles. The method is easy to use and provides some degree of quantitative evaluation. At present there are various different verbal analog scales in use, in which an example of intensity is given for each point:

- No pain.
- Pain I can ignore.
- Pain I cannot ignore, but that does not prevent me from living normally; that is, I am able to do what I want to do in spite of the pain.

- Pain that makes it difficult to concentrate on a task, like reading a book.
- Pain that interferes with most of my actions.
- Pain so severe that I can think of nothing else and cannot concentrate on anything else at all.
- Unbearable pain, for which I need medical help without delay.

Another technique is to furnish patients with small portable computers that they carry around with them and feed information into about the intensity of their pain at intervals during the day. This means that the intensity of the pain can be registered over a period of time.

In ordinary clinical practice one can usually obtain a good impression of the intensity and consequences of the pain by asking how far it affects the patient's daily life:

Does the pain interfere with ordinary tasks?
Does it prevent sleep?
Does it occupy the patient's thoughts to the exclusion of everything else?

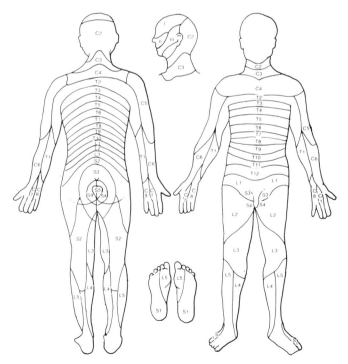

FIGURE 14. Dermatome chart.

FACTORS THAT AGGRAVATE
OR ALLEVIATE PAIN

Is the pain related to movement?
Is it worse after meals?
Does it improve after a bowel movement?

Finding the factors that influence the pain helps to determine the type of pain and the correct treatment for the particular patient.

VARIATIONS IN PAIN OVER TIME

Is the pain constant all the time?
Does it vary in intensity?
Does the patient have pain-free periods?

Sometimes it can be useful to draw up a timetable of when the various pains arise, when they feel worse, and so on, including all the variations over a 24-hour period.

THE PATIENT'S RESPONSE TO PREVIOUS
PAIN TREATMENT

An exact list should be obtained of all the medicines taken by the patient, with the doses, times, and so forth. If the patient's history shows that the pain has previously responded well to codeine, it is fairly certain that morphine and other opiates will have a good effect. If the pain has not responded at all to recommended analgesic treatment, a different approach should be tried. Usually a few questions will reveal that the analgesic has been prescribed in too small doses at too long intervals.

EFFECT OF EMOTIONAL, SOCIAL,
AND EXISTENTIAL (SPIRITUAL) FACTORS
ON THE PATIENT'S EXPERIENCE OF PAIN

These factors, as already mentioned, play a central role in the patient's experience of pain. It has been found again and again that help with psychological, social, and/or existential or spiritual problems has also brought relief from pain.

Pain that does not respond at all to ordinary treatment may depend to a considerable extent on these factors. Treatment in such cases should include consultation with other experts on such problems. The social consequences of the pain for the patient should not be neglected either—does it provide a secondary reward in the form of increased attention from family or nursing staff, or does it isolate the patient socially?

The impressions of the patient's family and of colleagues and nursing staff are often helpful in determining the nature of the pain.

ETIOLOGY OF PAIN

Studies have shown that patients with cancer often suffer from several different kinds of pain at the same time. A patient with metastasis to the spine may have increased muscular tension in the surrounding area because of the pain and will then have muscular pains as well. A patient who is being treated with a centrally active analgesic without accompanying doses of laxative may have stomach pains caused by constipation, and so on (see Table 2 on page 45).

Different types of pain should thus be considered and treated separately. In the above examples, it would be right to increase the dose of analgesic for the patient with increased pain caused by spinal metastasis, but this would be contraindicated for the patient with constipation pains, because such analgesics tend to aggravate constipation.

PAIN NOT DUE TO A NEOPLASM

We sometimes tend to forget that cancer patients may also have benign diseases. Pain in the back is not necessarily due to metastasis; a cancer patient can also suffer from lumbago. There is a wealth of examples of inadequate or inaccurate diagnoses of diseases accompanying cancer, resulting, of course, in incorrect treatment.

Cancer patients have a high frequency of pain in the musculoskeletal system, partly because they suffer so much from anxiety and insecurity, which often lead to muscular tension.

The pain may also be secondary to the pain of the cancer, or it may result from being bedridden. A correct diagnosis of the musculoskeletal pain can save the patient from having to take higher doses of morphine. An injection of a local anesthetic in a trigger point or tendon attachment can in many cases bring substantial relief, obviating the need for stronger analgesics.

Cancer patients often suffer from tension headaches and dyspepsia.

PAIN DUE TO A NEOPLASM

Skeletal Metastasis

Skeletal metastases are among the most common types of metastasis and are the cause of pain in about 50% of all cancer patients whose pain is due to their tumor. Skeletal metastasis is most common in connection with myeloma and malignant melanoma and cancer of the breast, lung, prostate, kidneys, and thyroid gland. The most common sites are the vertebrae, pelvis, and proximally in the limbs.

There is no clear correlation between the size of the metastasis and the pain. Small metastases sometimes cause severe pain, and large ones may cause less. The pain is usually chronic, deep-seated, and aching (protopathic). It is often aggravated by movement and by putting weight on the affected part. Tenderness is usually evident on direct palpation or indirectly on movement of the affected structures. When compression or fracture is present the pain is sharp, stabbing, and related to movement (epicritic). Skeletal metastasis may also be associated with infiltration in neighboring soft tissue and nerve tissue. Secondary muscular spasms often occur.

A supplementary examination is usually necessary, beginning with an X-ray examination, which reveals 50–75% of skeletal metastases. Metastases at the base of the skull and in the vertebrae (especially the seventh cervical to the first thoracic) and the sacrum can be difficult to see on X-rays, however. Scintigraphy is a more sensitive method, which allows the detection of 90% of skeletal metastases, often months before they can be seen on an X-ray. The drawbacks are that it may give false positive results (e.g. in the case of osteoporosis and fractures), and it is not a reliable indicator of skeletal metastasis in previously irradiated areas. But although skeletal metastasis is almost always revealed by one of these methods, it cannot be excluded as a diagnosis in cases where the findings are negative but the patient still has pains in the bone. Retroperitoneal and paravertebral metastases and metastases in the pelvis and the base of the skull may only be visible by computed tomography. Laboratory tests in the form of acid or alkaline phosphatases may also be necessary.

Both tumor cells and osteoclasts resorb bone and lead to areas of osteolysis. Many efforts have been made to try to discover the chemical substances that induce osteolysis, and there is strong evidence that prostaglandin E_2 is involved. This opens up a number of interesting treatment possibilities. Animal experiments and in vitro experiments with human cancer cells have shown that prostaglandin inhibitors (e.g., aspirin) can reduce osteolytic activity. We also know that prostaglandin E_2 lowers the pain threshold peripherally. Thus peripherally active analgesics (nonsteroidal anti-inflammatory drugs, or NSAIDs) should theoretically relieve the pain of skeletal metastasis, and clinical experience has confirmed this. Glucocorticosteroids inhibit prostaglandin synthesis at an earlier stage than NSAIDs, and this, together with the antiedema effect of the steroid component, makes them a good alternative in the treatment of pain from skeletal metastasis (see Fig. 24). Radiotherapy is also very effective.

The various treatments for the relief of pain from skeletal metastasis are as follows: NSAIDs, glucocorticosteroids, radiotherapy, analgesics, surgical fixation. The methods of treatment will be discussed in detail in Chapter 10.

Compression and/or Infiltration of Nerves

Compression and/or infiltration of the nerves is the cause of pain in about 25% of cases where pain is directly due to the tumor.

Compression of Nerves

The pain may be either deep-seated and aching or superficial and burning (see p. 28). It is felt at the site of compression and/or throughout the area supplied by the nerve. It may be constant or intermittent, and it often occurs long before any sensory or motor deficits become evident. The area of innervation is frequently tender when palpated. Thus distal pathology, and not proximal nerve compression, may appear to be the cause of the pain, until the growing tumor gives rise to characteristic sensory and motor deficits. Pains due to compression of the nerves caused by a pathological fracture may be sharp, tearing, and related to movement.

A small percentage of cancer patients experience compression of the spinal cord or the cauda equina, usually because of metastasis to the vertebral body or infiltration of the intervertebral foramina. Occasionally this is caused directly by intramedullary metastasis. Pain is the most common symptom of compression of the medulla and it is usually added to the pain caused by the spinal metastasis. With compression, the pain is bilateral and does not follow dermatomes. If the compression affects the roots of nerves leading out of the spine to any great extent, the pain will be radiating, either unilaterally or bilaterally, Such pains usually correspond to dermatomes. The pains are either sharp, stabbing, and radiating, or they feel like tight bands around the body or limbs. The patient may also have sensory or motor deficits and/or disturbed function of the bladder or bowels (incontinence).

Infiltration of Nerves

Pain caused by direct tumor infiltration of nerve structures is often burning and superficial. The patient may have allodynia (see p. 29) and hyperpathia. The pain in the affected nerves may be caused by substances secreted by the tumor, which may initiate impulses in the nerve fibers. The nature of these substances is not known. Another cause of pain is that the injured nerve structures regenerate and form sprouts. (This mechanism is described in Chapter 1, p. 7) This process usually makes the nerve fibers hypersensitive to norepinephrine and mechanical influences.

It is common for the body's largest nerve plexuses, like the brachial or the lumbosacral plexus, to be affected. A dermatome chart is a good aid to diagnosis in such cases, although it is important to realize that usually the nerves are only partly affected, so that the damage does not entirely correspond to the dematome (see Fig. 14).

Meningeal carcinomatosis is usually painful. Approximately half the patients suffer from headaches, usually frontal, and many also from increased intracranial pressure. Pains in the back are also frequent, usually in the lumbosacral area, and in many cases the pain radiates down the legs because the roots of the nerves are affected.

Polyradiculoneuropathy

Polyradiculoneuropathy, which may be a paraneoplastic syndrome due to a distant effect of a tumor, can give rise in some patient to symptoms of nerve injury, with or without pain. This may occur several months before the primary tumor gives any symptoms. The neurological deficits are often reversible if the primary cancer is treated, and the pain will then diminish.

The following treatments for compression and/or infiltration of the nerves are available:

Glucocorticosteroids
Analgesics
Antiepileptic drugs
Antidepressants
Nerve blocks (somatic and sympathetic)
Radiotherapy
Neurosurgery

Infiltration of Hollow Organs or Excretory Ducts from Abdominal Organs

Infiltrative growth in hollow organs or excretory ducts from abdominal organs may manifest itself as colic or gastrointestinal obstruction. This is usually a complication of gastrointestinal cancer or cancer of the ovaries with spread to the peritoneum. Sometimes an "attack of gallstones" may have a malignant etiology and ureteral colic may be caused by blood clots from a kidney tumor.

The following treatments are available:

Surgery
Radiotherapy
Cytostatic drugs
Analgesics
Antiemetics
Anticholinergics

Stretching of the Capsules Surrounding Internal Organs

Metastases in the liver, cancer of the pancreas, hypernephroma, and so on cause stretching of the capsule, although in a large number of cases the tumor grows without causing pain. When pain does occur, it is constant, deep-seated, and aching. It is located in the area of the affected organ and is often accompanied by referred pain.

Abdominal palpation may reveal the etiology of the pain, but further examination is usually necessary by X-rays (and sometimes computed tomography), a liver scan, and ultrasound.

Tumors in the lungs are usually painless unless they grow into the chest wall or obstruct bronchi or blood vessels. Mediastinal tumors can cause pain in the middle of the chest, which may resemble the characteristic pains of heart disease.

The following treatments are available:

Glucocorticosteroids
NSAIDs
Analgesics
Radiotherapy
Cytostatic drugs, if necessary intra-arterial infusion
Surgery

Compression and/or Infiltration of Blood and Lymph Vessels

Compression and/or infiltration of blood vessels can lead to venostasis with peripheral edema and/or ischemia. Edema causes stretching of fasciae and other sensitive structures. The pain is deep-seated, aching, and diffuse. Edema of the nerves can also cause neuralgia. Particularly painful and uncomfortable conditions are Stokes' disease, with infiltration/occlusion in the vena cava superior, edema of the upper limbs due to breast cancer, edema of the lower limbs due to cancer in the pelvis, and headache with obstruction of the venous drainage from the head. Ischemia is well known to be extremely painful.

The following treatments are available:

Surgery
Radiotherapy
High Doses of glucocorticosteroids
Diuretics
Analgesics
Use of an anti-edema pulsator
Maintenance of the affected limb higher than the heart

Infiltration of Soft Tissue

Some soft-tissue tumors may become quite large before they cause any pain, and in such cases there is no doubt where the pain is coming from, since the tumor can be palpated. In other cases pain occurs earlier, especially if the tumor causes stretching of fasciae, tendons, periosteum, etc. Soft tissue infiltration in the extremities often causes pain on movement. The pain is usually deep-seated and aching.

Ulcerating tumors on the skin and mucous membranes can be painful. Here the patient may have both deep-seated, aching pain and more superficial, burning pain. A certain degree of inflammation is always present, and bacterial or fungal infection is a common complication.

The following treatments are available:

Radiation
Surgery
Glucocorticosteroids
Antibiotics/Antimycotics
Analgesics
Local treatment of the wound

Headache Due to Increased Intracranial Pressure

Headaches from increased intracranial pressure are often diffuse but may be located directly over the tumor or be mostly unilateral. The headache is often aggravated by increased intra-abdominal pressure (straining) and sometimes by lying down (morning headache). Gagging and vomiting, frequently without nausea, are often early symptoms. The syndrome often gives rise to neurological deficits, involving paresis or loss of sensibility, and can affect vision or hearing. Marked psychological changes may occur. Papillary stasis is a late sign of a supratentorial tumor. In infratentorial tumors, on the other hand, the increased pressure on the brain is due to obstructed drainage of the cerebrospinal fluid. A little over half the number of intracranial tumors are metastases, and these usually give rise to less pronounced symptoms than primary central nervous system tumors.

The following treatments are available:

Surgery
Radiation
Glucocorticosteriods
Analgesics

PAIN DUE TO CANCER TREATMENT

About 20% of cancer patients who suffer from pain do so because of the treatment of their disease.

Pain Following Surgery

Injury to Nerves

In major surgery it is impossible to avoid severing nerves. During regeneration small sprouts and neuromas, which can be hypersensitive to touch and to norepinephrine (see Chapter 1, p. 7), often form. Constant pain may arise in the area of sensory deficit 1 to 2 months after the operation.

Emotional stress increases the pain, probably because of increased secretion of norepinephrine. Every now and then severe, stabbing pains of short duration occur, triggered by touch or movement in the affected part. They may be so distressing that the patient will do almost anything to get rid of them. This type of pain is most usual after thoracotomy, mastectomy, and radical neck dissection.

Pain Following Thoracotomy

The patient may have constant pain in the area supplied by the intercostal nerves in the scar tissue. This often takes the form of dysesthesia with hyperesthesia in the surrounding area. Because movement often provokes the pain, patients tend to avoid moving their arms, which can result in a frozen shoulder with accompanying atrophy of the arm. Since such pains may be due to tumor growth, metastasis should be excluded by X-rays, computed tomography, or biopsy.

Pain Following Mastectomy

Mastectomy can give rise to several pain syndromes.

Acute/subacute postmastectomy pain is usually due to injury to the intercostobrachial nerve during the operation. The patient often feels a burning, constricting pain in the lateral wall of the thorax, the axilla, and the inside upper arm. There may be allodynia and hyperesthesia. The pain is aggravated by cold weather and movement of the arm, so that these patients have a tendency to develop frozen shoulder. This pain condition may become chronic, although in the majority of cases it lasts for less than 6 months.

Chronic nonmalignant postmastectomy pain is a chronic pain condition that begins a relatively short time after the mastectomy. The patient feels a burning pain in the front of the thorax, with a distribution that cannot be explained by a nerve injury. The pain is usually aggravated by the touch of clothes or the breast prosthesis, but normally does not respond to the pressure of a stethoscope. There is no tenderness in the sternum or ribs, but there are often trigger points in the pain area. This pain is probably largely conditioned by social and psychological factors. Many of these patients are emotionally labile and subject to periods of depression. The pain often has considerable social consequences, and many of these patients gradually develop a chronic pain syndrome, which dominates their lives.

The differential diagnosis in these two conditions is primarily tumor growth, and a thorough and complete investigation of the pain is therefore essential.

Pain Following Radical Neck Dissection

The mechanism behind the type of pain that can follow radical neck dissection is probably damage to nervous tissue. Usually it is characterized by burning pains in the area of loss of sensibility. Dysesthesia and sudden, intermittent pains also occur. Some of these patients also have pains that radiate out to the shoulder and down the arm on the same side.

The following treatments are available for pain due to nerve injury:

Antidepressants
Antiepileptic drugs
Transcutaneous electric nerve stimulation (TENS)
Repeated injections of local anesthetics at painful sites (neuromas) and, if
    necessary, glucocorticosteroids
Nerve blocks (somatic and sympathetic)
Cryoanalgesia
Analgesics

Pain Following Amputation

Pain may occur after amputation either in the stump or in the form of phantom pains, that is, pains that feel as though they come from the missing limb. Most patients have pains in the stump after the operation, but these generally recede and after 6 months are present in less than 10% of patients. Pains in the stump are of all kinds, ranging from aches to dysesthesia and shooting pains. Sometimes they are due to scar tissue and adhesions, sometimes to pressure on a neuroma.

Phantom pains are usually perceived as coming from the periphery of the lost limb. They often feel as if they are produced by pressing and squeezing, but they can also be stabbing and radiating. Patients who experienced a lot of pain before the amputation are predisposed to phantom pains, which often resemble the preoperative pain. Phantom pains are occasionally due to pressure on a neuroma.

The following treatments are available:

TENS
Antiepileptic drugs and/or antidepressants
Nerve blocks (somatic and sympathetic)
Analgesics
Reoperation
Neurosurgery

Adhesions

These may develop several months after an operation, especially in the abdomen. The intestinal wall may adhere to the peritoneum or to another part of the intestine, or the intestine may become constricted. The patient experiences severe colic, with pains that come and go, depending among other things on the intestinal contents. The pain from adhesions may be very distressing and may become worse with time.

The following treatments are available:

Reoperation
Analgesics
Anticholinergics

Pain Following Chemotherapy

Painful polyradiculoneuropathy. Painful polyradiculoneuropathy may arise after treatment with *Vinca* alkaloids (like vincristine or vinblastine) or cisplatin. The pain often takes the form of "burning feet." It usually stops some time after the medication has been discontinued but can occasionally last for months or years.

The following treatments are available for long-term symptoms:

Antidepressants
Sympathetic block with intravenous guanethidine
TENS

Aseptic necrosis of the caput femoris or caput humeri may occur after treatment with steroids or other cytostatic drugs. It should be treated surgically if possible.

Steroid pseudorheumatism can occur after patients have discontinued steroid medication. Patients suffer from diffuse pain in the muscles and joints, and their general health is affected. The condition improves if steroid therapy is resumed.

Herpes Zoster (Shingles) and Postherpetic Neuralgia

Patients with cancer and those undergoing treatment with cytostatic and immunosuppressive drugs have an increased incidence of herpes zoster.

In acute herpes zoster, the patient first feels pain along the course of one or more nerves. This is followed by the eruption of vesicles, which dry up after some time. The pain is described as continuous and aching or burning, with paroxysms of shooting or lancinating pain, the latter often triggered by touch or movement of the skin in the affected dermatome. Many patients complain of itching in the painful area. The affected dermatomes are often hyperesthetic, and the patient has allodynia. Because patients try to avoid moving the affected part, they will often have secondary muscular or skeletal pain. The acute attack may last for several weeks or, where there is a poorly functioning immune system, for several months.

Many of these patients, especially older people, develop postherpetic neuralgia. The pain resembles that of the acute attack, with continuous burning, aching pain interspersed with paroxysms of shooting, radiating pains. The patients often have allodynia and hyperpathia. This pain condition is often accompanied by depressive symptoms, sleep disturbances, anorexia, and frequently considerable changes in personality and life-style. Many of these patients develop a chronic pain syndrome.

The following treatments are available for acute herpes zoster:

Acyclovir (especially for patients treated with immunosuppressive drugs)
Steroids (for patients with a normal immune system)
Analgesics
Nerve block during the acute stage

Treatments for postherpetic neuralgia:

TENS
Antidepressants (amitriptyline)
Antiepileptic drugs
Repeated subcutaneous injections of local anesthetic and steroids in the painful area
Sometimes opioid analgesics

Pain Following Radiotherapy

Local edema, which sometimes causes pain, can occur during the acute phase of radiotherapy and just afterward. Some time afterward, fibrosis begins in the irradiated area and continues for a considerable period, during which the tissue gradually shrinks, sometimes causing compression of nerves and other structures. Radiation can also lead to demyelination of nerve tissue.

The most common pain conditions after radiotherapy are fibrosis of the brachial and lumbosacral plexuses. It is important, but difficult, to distinguish pain caused by radiation fibrosis from pain caused by local recurrence of the cancer. Even computed tomography may not distinguish the two, and surgical exploration may be necessary.

Both radiation fibrosis and recurrence of the cancer can give rise to pain, paresthesia, and numbness, which occur much earlier than paresis. The pain is often a continuous ache, sometimes a burning pain. Hyperesthesia and lancinating pain are rare. The pain becomes worse with time. The interval between the end of the treatment and the start of the pain ranges from 2 months to 20 years. Very severe pain is an indication of metastasizing cancer, and cancer also leads to a higher frequency of Horner's syndrome and symptoms in the lower part of the plexus brachialis. When radiation is the cause, there is a higher frequency of lymphedema in the arm.

Irradiation of the abdomen can give rise to colic and chronic diarrhea because of atrophy and fibrosis of the intestine.

The following treatments are available:

Glucocorticosteroids
TENS

Analgesics
Antidepressants
Antiepileptic drugs
Nerve blocks

Pain due to Inactivity and Confinement to Bed

As the cancer progresses, the patient becomes gradually weaker and is usually bedridden toward the end. This sometimes leads to pressure sores, which can be very painful, and to pain in muscles and bones, due to strain on the muscles and ligaments, muscular spasms with trigger points, and inactivity osteoporosis. Confinement to bed also predisposes to thrombosis and embolism, and when a patient has acute pain in the chest and there is no evidence of metastasis to the lung or mediastinum, lung embolism should be suspected.

The following treatments are available:

Regular changes of position in bed
Trigger point treatment, e.g., injections
Activation of the patient, where possible
Analgesics
TENS

TABLE 2. Etiology of Pain in Cancer Patients

Pain not due to the neoplasm
Pain due to the neoplasm
  Skeletal metastasis
  Compression/infiltration of nerves
  Infiltrative growth in hollow organs or excretory ducts from abdominal organs
  Stretching of the capsules around internal organs
  Compression/infiltration of blood vessels
  Soft-tissue infiltration
  Headache caused by increased intracranial pressure
Pain due to cancer treatment
  Pain following surgery
  Pain following chemotherapy
  Pain following radiotherapy
  Pain due to inactivity and confinement to bed.

3

Principles
of Treatment

As we have already discussed, chronic pain is qualitatively different from acute pain, and its treatment should naturally be qualitatively different from the treatment of acute pain.

When a patient has an incurable cancer, it is essential that the physician and nursing staff do not adopt a resigned attitude. The patient has the right to receive active help for pain and other symptoms as they arise. People with a poor prognosis should not be dismissed as being merely "in need of nursing"; proper treatment and sensitive care—that is, appropriate pain treatment, increased mobility, and good psychosocial care—given during this phase make a great difference to the quality of life.

PRINCIPLES OF TREATMENT

1. A thorough assessment of the pain condition is essential for correct treatment.
2. The therapeutic environment and the relationship between physician and patient are crucial.
3. The treatment must be well planned.
4. The patient must be kept informed and encouraged to participate actively in the treatment.
5. The patient should *not* be encouraged to put up with the pain for as long as possible.

6. Chronic pain requires continuous and prophylactic treatment.
7. Persistent pain should be treated at regular intervals and not "as required" (pro re nata, p.r.n.).
8. Analgesics should be given orally as far as possible.
9 Sufficiently large doses should be prescribed.
10. The assessment of pain and the response to treatment should be continually monitored.

A THOROUGH ASSESSMENT OF THE PAIN CONDITION IS ESSENTIAL FOR CORRECT TREATMENT

It is important to remember that the assessment of a pain should include both the sensory and the psychological components. Different types of pain respond differently to analgesics, so a correct diagnosis is a prerequisite for effective pain relief.

THE THERAPEUTIC ENVIRONMENT AND THE RELATIONSHIP BETWEEN PHYSICIAN AND PATIENT ARE CRUCIAL

The process of assessment creates a relationship between physician and patient that strongly affects the results of the treatment. A number of studies have shown that a secure, warm, and friendly environment can greatly reduce the consumption of analgesics. This is not surprising when one considers how strongly psychological factors influence the endogenous pain-inhibiting mechanisms. Everyone who comes in contact with a patient can thus significantly contribute to relieving the pain.

THE TREATMENT MUST BE WELL PLANNED

Other methods of treatment such as radiation or nerve blocks should be considered before large doses of strong analgesics are started. All the available reversible techniques should be tried before any of the irreversible ones are attempted (phenol block, neurosurgery, etc.).

All treatment takes time, and it is unwise to promise the patient relief within the first day or so. It should be explained that an individual therapeutic regimen suitable for the patient's needs is being worked out. There are good grounds for optimism in the treatment of pain, and one can generally promise an improvement within a few days. The first goal is to ensure pain relief at night, so that the patient can sleep and gather strength for the following day. The next goal should be relief at rest during the day, and finally, if possible, painless movement.

THE PATIENT MUST BE KEPT INFORMED
AND ENCOURAGED TO PARTICIPATE
ACTIVELY IN THE TREATMENT

It is important to provide patients with written information about their treatment, especially when they are being treated outside an institution. The information should include the purpose of the medicines and when they should be taken.

Example Patient: John Smith

Before breakfast	Morphine mixture (for pain)	10 ml
At breakfast	Prednisolone (for pain, stimulates the appetite)	2 tablets
10 a.m.	Morphine mixture	10 ml
	Peri-Colase (laxative)	1 tablet
2 p.m.	Morphine mixture	10 ml
6 p.m.	Morphine mixture	10 ml
	Peri-Colace	1 tablet
8 p.m.	Saroten (sleeping pill, improves mood)	2 tablets
At bedtime	Morphine mixture	10 ml
For pain during the night	Morphine mixture	10 ml
If the pain gets worse	Increase the mixture dose to	15 ml

If case of new or aggravated symptoms, call me at one of the following numbers, 50 60 50 (work) or 54 97 88 (home).
Next appointment: Friday, December 13.

The patient should be told beforehand of the most common side effects of the treatment (especially sedation) and of what can be done to counteract them. Side effects tend to disappear gradually, but prior information about them often determines whether or not a patient continues with the treatment.

THE PATIENT SHOULD
NOT BE ENCOURAGED TO PUT UP WITH
THE PAIN FOR AS LONG AS POSSIBLE

Pain should be treated as soon as it begins to become a problem. The patient should become used to receiving help for the pain. With chronic pain, the peripheral pain threshold may be lowered and the supply of endorphins in the central nervous system also appears to become diminished. One of the most common mistakes in pain conditions is to wait too long before starting treatment, because of fear that the drugs will gradually become less effective. In fact, this does not happen (see p. 86). If the treatment is started early it is easier to keep the pain at bay during all subsequent phases of the disease.

CHRONIC PAIN REQUIRES CONTINUOUS AND PROPHYLACTIC TREATMENT

Chronic pain is far too often treated as if it were an acute attack, each time the dose of analgesic ceases to take effect. The pain should not be allowed to return before the next dose is taken. Pain should thus be treated in advance, that is, prophylactically. This means that:

PERSISTENT PAIN SHOULD BE TREATED AT REGULAR INTERVALS AND NOT "AS REQUIRED" (PRO RE NATA, P.R.N.)

If pain is treated regularly, patients have no need to fear its return (see Fig. 15). This gives them a sense of security and enables them to concentrate on other aspects of life. When analgesics are administered p.r.n., patients become very preoccupied by their pain, because they are responsible for relieving it themselves and have to ask for the next dose. In their anxiety to prevent the pain from returning, they will often tend to reduce the intervals between doses and ask for higher and higher doses. This can lead to a higher consumption of analgesics than among those who follow a regular timetable. It is easier to prevent pain than to treat a pain already present, and prophylactic doses do not usually need to be as high.

ANALGESICS SHOULD BE GIVEN ORALLY AS FAR AS POSSIBLE

Another common mistake is to begin giving injections of analgesics too early. Studies have shown that about 85% of patients can take drugs orally until the last few days before death.

Oral administration gives a more level concentration in serum and consequently more constant relief from pain (see Fig. 16). An injection leads to a rapid peak in serum concentration and the pain-relieving effect rapidly recedes. Repeated injections also represent a problem in themselves. An analgesic in liquid form has some advantages over a tablet. The mixture is easier to swallow and the dose can be increased without increasing the volume. Many patients, however, dislike the taste of the mixture and prefer to take tablets.

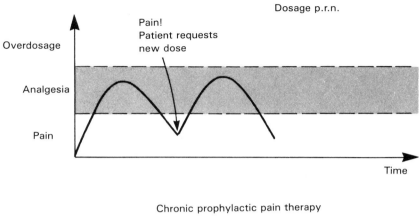

Dosage p.r.n.

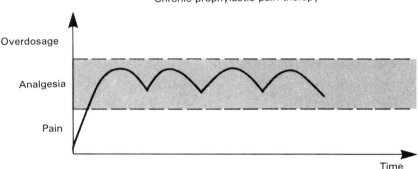

Chronic prophylactic pain therapy

FIGURE 15. Diagram of two different principles for the dosage of analgesics. (Adapted from R. Twycross, *Acta Anaestl. Scand.* 26 (Suppl. 74):83–90, 1982.)

SUFFICIENTLY LARGE DOSES SHOULD BE PRESCRIBED

The doses recommended in the *Physicians' Desk Reference* for strong analgesics are often based on experience with postoperative pain or other acute conditions. They have been shown to be quite inadequate for treating chronic cancer pain, for which the dose often has to be increased many times to obtain the desired effect. Considerable pharmacological knowledge is needed to be able to judge which drugs can safely be given in large doses and which will give serious side effects and/or cumulative effects at high doses.

Tolerance is said to develop when the use of a drug over a long period leads to the dose having to be increased in order to achieve the same effect as before. All opioids have this property. The development of tolerance does not mean that the patient has become "dependent" of "addicted"; it is a normal biochemical process. Tolerance develops sooner with parenteral than with oral treatment. In practice, this is not a problem as regards the

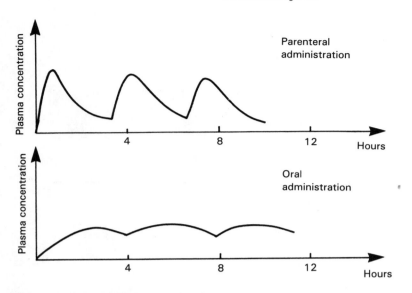

FIGURE 16. Concentration of morphine in serum after parenteral and oral administration.

treatment of pain in cancer patients, because the dose can be increased and the patient obtain relief without a corresponding increase in the frequency of side effects. In other words, the drug does not lose its analgesic effect.

As a result of public interest in drug addiction and the strict control over the prescription of strong opioids, the consumption of strong analgesics by ambulant patients was substantially reduced during the 1970s. This undoubtedly had many positive effects, but it equally certainly caused problems for patients with chronic cancer pain who required opioid treatment. During the last few years, however, the supply of strong analgesics to cancer patients has increased considerably.

Several studies have been carried out on the risk of drug addiction (psychological addiction, euphomania) among cancer patients treated according to the principles mentioned above. They conclude that the risk is insignificant. It is greater when the treatment is given p.r.n., that is, if the patient's anxiety about the pain is allowed to dominate the treatment. Parenteral treatment is also thought to be more likely to create addiction than oral treatment. As a general rule, drug addiction is not a problem in the treatment of pain in cancer patients and patients with a poor life expectancy.

THE ASSESSMENT OF PAIN AND THE RESPONSE TO TREATMENT SHOULD BE CONTINUALLY MONITORED

Regular contact with the patient is important. New symptoms may arise that require changes in dosage or a different method of treatment. The treatment of persistent pain is a continuous process. The difference between good treatment and bad lies in how far the patient is followed up. It is rare to find an effective and appropriate method of treating the pain at the first attempt, and it is normal to try out increased doses and new methods.

The methods used to treat pain and other symptoms of cancer are of two kinds: those that give symptomatic relief from pain and those that remove or reduce the tumor and thus treat the cause of the pain. The following methods belong to the first group:

Drugs
Nerve blocks
Neurosurgery
Transcutaneous electrical nerve stimulation (TENS)
Acupuncture

Methods that remove or reduce the tumor include the following:

Surgery
Radiotherapy
Cytostatic drugs
Endocrine therapy

The discussion of drugs will be comprehensive and detailed, since they are the basis of most treatments. The other methods will be briefly described, and the emphasis will be on the indications for referral to specialists in oncology, neurosurgery, or anesthesiology.

Until recently, survival time was the only important criterion used in measuring the efficiency of methods for treating cancer. A method that did not prolong survival was regarded as ineffective. Fortunately, there is now a growing interest in methods that improve the quality of life and do not merely prolong it. When used properly, such methods can considerably increase a patient's well-being and to a large extent provide relief from pain.

PART II

METHODS OF TREATING PAIN AND OTHER CANCER-RELATED SYMPTOMS

4

A Short
Pharmacological
Survey

A knowledge of the pharmacology of analgesics is essential for an effective and rational treatment of pain in cancer. I shall start with a brief recapitulation of the principles of pharmacokinetics. This process can be divided into the following stages: absorption, distribution (in the body), biotransformation (metabolism, degradation), and elimination/excretion.

ABSORPTION

The absorption of a drug depends on the method of administration.

Intravenous administration causes no problems of absorption. The effect is rapid, but there is a risk of side effects caused by an excessively high concentration in serum if the drug is injected too rapidly.

Intramuscular administration usually leads to good absorption, although certain drugs, like the benzodiazepine group, are absorbed very erratically. Intramuscular administration involves fewer risks than intravenous injection, but it can be painful.

Subcutaneous administration leads to a slower and sometimes more erratic rate of absorption than the two previous methods, since the absorption depends on the supply of blood to the area. Certain drugs can cause local inflammation or necrosis when administered in this way.

Rectal administration is useful if there is nausea or vomiting, but the absorption may be erratic and slow. It is also hindered if the rectum is full of feces, and some patients react with a defecation reflex and eject the suppository or suspension.

Sublingual administration causes rapid absorption and the drug enters the systemic circulation directly without having to pass through the liver. However, many drugs are not effectively absorbed sublingually. If the patient swallows spit, of course, the administration is in fact oral, and some drugs, like buprenorphine, are thereby inactivated.

Oral administration is usually the best method and results in the most even concentrations in serum. The absorption can be retarded if the drug is taken in conjunction with food, but if the drug has a high first-pass metabolism the food intake can actually increase its bioavailability. The method can give rise to local irritation in the gastrointestinal tract and is not suitable for patients with severe nausea and vomiting. Absorption through the mucous membrane of the stomach and intestines seldom causes any difficulties with the drugs discussed below and will not be treated in any detail in this book.

FIRST-PASS METABOLISM

All drugs that are absorbed from the intestines have to pass through the intestinal mucosa and the liver in order to enter the systemic circulation. Part of the dose is metabolized during this first passage through the intestinal wall and the liver and therefore does not reach the target organ. This is called the first-pass metabolism and it is dose dependent, since small doses may be completely degraded. The enzyme systems in the liver have a limited capacity, however, and if it is exceeded by a high enough dosage, the remainder of the drug passes unchanged through the liver. In such cases a small increase in the dose can give rise to a large increase in the concentration in plasma. Drugs with a substantial first-pass metabolism are the opiates, tricyclic antidepressants, some antiepileptics, and beta-blockers. There are great individual differences.

BIOAVAILABILITY

The plasma concentration over time, signified by the area under the curve (AUC), may be much smaller after oral ingestion than after intravenous injection (see Fig. 17). Bioavailability is defined as

$$\frac{\text{AUC orally}}{\text{AUC intravenously}} \times 100$$

and is expressed as a percentage. Reduced bioavailability is often due to a sizable first-pass metabolism through the liver.

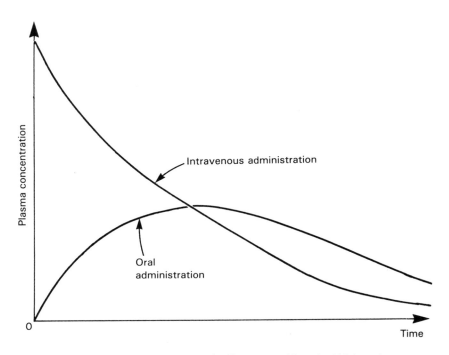

$$\text{Bioavailability} = \frac{\text{area under the curve with oral administration}}{\text{area under the curve with intravenous administration}}$$

FIGURE 17. Biological availability of a drug.

DISTRIBUTION IN THE BODY

After absorption and sometimes passage through the liver, the drug enters the systemic circulation and is distributed to the tissues. The distribution is governed by several factors, including blood supply to the tissues, plasma protein binding, binding to the tissue, and transport barriers (blood-brain barrier).

BLOOD SUPPLY TO THE TISSUES

About 15% of the minute volume of the heart at rest reaches the central nervous system, and much of the drug will therefore be transported along with it. Drugs that pass easily through the blood-brain barrier will therefore rapidly attain a high concentration in the central nervous system. The muscles receive about 20% of the minute volume of the heart and a corresponding proportion of the drug. Over 90% of administered morphine is found in the muscular tissue, and this is one of the reasons why elderly people, with their comparatively small muscular mass, are more sensitive to morphine.

PLASMA PROTEIN BINDING

Drugs with acidic groups (e.g., aspirinlike drugs) have a high binding affinity to albumin, while drugs like amitriptyline, chlorpromazine, and propranolol bind largely to lipoproteins and the acute-phase protein orosomucoid.

Only the free, unbound fraction of the drug is active. Plasma protein binding can therefore act as a depot and ensures a constant supply of the active fraction during the intervals between doses. If more than one drug with a high protein-binding capacity is administered, the protein-binding capacity of plasma protein may be exceeded, and a larger fraction may be liberated with a correspondingly greater effect. This presents few practical problems. The free fraction is increased in patients with hypoalbuminemia, uremia, and hepatic insufficiency, a fact that needs to be remembered in the treatment of debilitated cancer patients in order to avoid overdosing them.

BINDING TO TISSUE

Tissue often has a greater affinity for drugs than plasma proteins do because it contains a greater number and variety of binding sites. The binding is usually reversible and is in equilibrium with the concentration in blood. Fat-soluble substances have a great affinity for fatty tissue, which can function as a drug depot.

The pH of the tissue concerned also affects the action of the drug. At a low pH acidic drugs (such as aspirinlike drugs) are displaced from the plasma proteins, leading to larger free fractions that can enter the cells. These drugs thus have a greater effect at a low pH, which is often found in inflamed and cancerous tissue. The opposite is true of alkaline drugs.

TRANSPORT BARRIERS (BLOOD-BRAIN BARRIER)

Transport across the capillary membrane usually poses no problem, because drugs have low molecular weights. The blood-brain barrier, however, prevents free distribution to the central nervous system. Transport through the blood-brain barrier usually occurs in the form of nonionic diffusion, and fat-soluble molecules pass easily across it. Water-soluble molecules have difficulty in crossing, but chronic intake of such a drug can give rise to a high concentration in the central nervous system.

BIOTRANSFORMATION (METABOLISM AND DEGRADATION)

The chemical structure of a drug is altered by contact with various enzyme systems. Passage through the liver can convert an inactive drug (a prodrug) to the active substance. Examples of this are prednisone, which is converted to the active substance prednisolone, and codeine, which is to some extent converted to morphine. Most biotransformation consists in the conversion of active drugs to less active and/or inactive metabolites. The most usual chemical reactions involved are oxidation, reduction, and hydrolysis. Lipophilic drugs have to be made more water soluble in order to be excreted by the kidneys. To achieve this, the metabolite is conjugated to a water-soluble substance already found in the body, such as glucuronic acid (the most common), sulfuric acid, acetic acid, or glycine.

ELIMINATION (EXCRETION)

The most important path of elimination, quantitatively speaking, is the excretion of water-soluble inactive metabolites through the kidneys. A number of drugs are excreted in an unaltered state (nonmetabolized) through the kidneys, and many others are transformed to inactive metabolites. In the latter case the kidneys are essential for the effective elimination of active substances. Elimination also occurs, to a lesser extent, through the bile and feces.

PHARMACOKINETICS

Pharmacokinetics also comprises the quantitative description of these four qualitatively different processes.

To facilitate this, the body can be viewed in a simplified way. For a drug that is distributed rapidly and evenly to all parts of the body, the latter can be seen as a single fluid-filled compartment (one-compartment model). For drugs that reach one part of the body rapidly and others more slowly, the body can be thought of as consisting of two or more compartments (the two-compartment model).

In the two-compartment model the body consists of a central distribution compartment (including well-perfused organs like the heart or brain) and a peripheral distribution compartment (see Fig. 18). The drug is rapidly transported to the central compartment, in which the concentration declines fairly rapidly, partly because the drug is distributed throughout the larger peripheral compartment (e.g., the skeletal muscles, connective tissue, subcutaneous layer) and partly because it is metabolized and excreted. Gradually, the concentration in the peripheral compartment increases until an equilibrium is achieved with the central compartment. After this point the peripheral compartment functions as a depot. The drug can be eliminated from the peripheral compartment only via the central compartment, so that elimination takes place at different speeds from the two compartments. This is expressed on a logarithmic scale in Fig. 19.

If distribution to the peripheral compartment is slow, a single dose of a drug will have the same duration of action as it would if it were distrib-

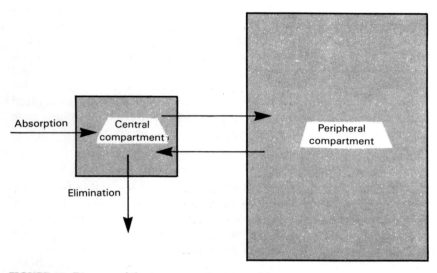

FIGURE 18. Diagram of the two-compartment model.

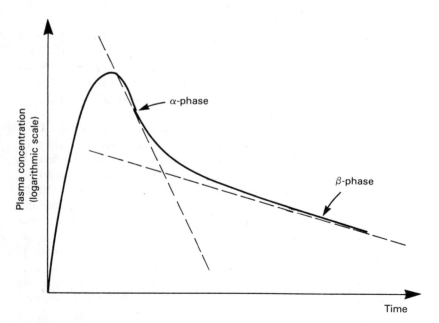

FIGURE 19. Plasma concentration curve for a drug distributed in the body according to the two-compartment model.

uted only to the central compartment. With long-term medication it is the elimination from the peripheral compartment that influences the time of action most, since the peripheral compartment then contains a large proportion of the drug. This applies, for example, to methadone and propoxyphene.

First-order elimination kinetics. This means that a certain *fraction* of a drug is eliminated per time unit. Elimination occurs rapidly at high concentrations. If the concentration is reduced by half, the speed of elimination diminishes correspondingly, but the eliminated fraction remains constant (see Fig. 20).

When this is expressed as a logarithmic curve, the result is a straight line, as shown in Fig. 21. When the elimination is rapid the curve drops steeply, and if elimination slows down the curve flattens out correspondingly.

Zero-order elimination kinetics. In such cases a *constant amount* of the drug is eliminated irrespective of the amount remaining in the body (see Fig. 22). This happens if the enzyme system metabolizing the drug is saturated and therefore breaks down only a certain amount however much it is supplied with. First-order elimination thus presupposes a certain amount of available enzyme capacity. With high doses a first-order elimination can become zero order if the enzyme system becomes saturated. It will then take longer than usual for the body to excrete the drug, and even a small increase in dose can produce a toxic concentration. This can occur with, for example, aspirin and phenytoin.

Half-life ($T_{1/2}$). The half-life is the time taken for the concentration in the distribution compartment to be halved. In practice, the concentration

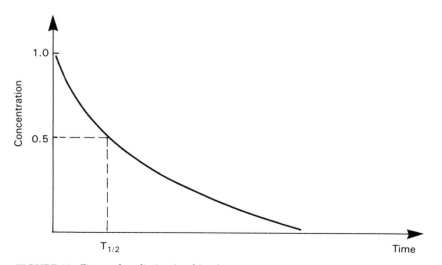

FIGURE 20. First-order elimination kinetics.

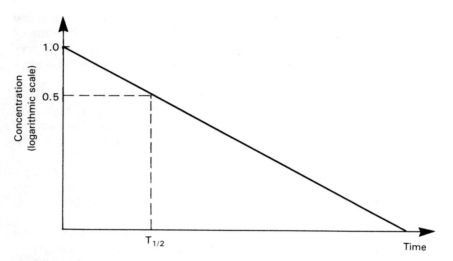

FIGURE 21. First-order elimination kinetics with the ordinate representing a logarithmic scale.

in serum is often used to estimate the half-life. The half-life thus represents the length of time between the peak concentration of the drug in serum until this concentration has been halved. In first-order kinetics the half-life is always constant, while in zero-order kinetics it depends on the amount of the drug administered. In the one-compartment model there is one half-life, but drugs whose mode of distribution follows the two-

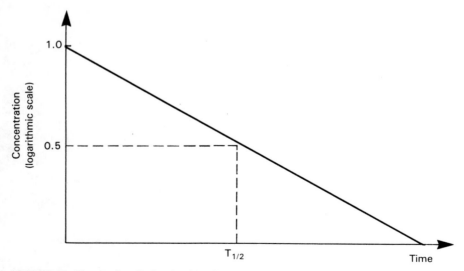

FIGURE 22. Zero-order elimination kinetics.

compartment model have two half-lives, one in the alpha phase and one in the beta phase, corresponding to the central and peripheral compartments, respectively (see Fig. 19).

Apparent volume of distribution (V_d). This is calculated according to the following formula:

$$V_d = \frac{\text{amount of drug in the body}}{\text{concentration in plasma}}$$

The apparent volume of distribution expresses the proportions of the drug present in plasma and tissue, respectively. A large apparent distribution volume indicates that most of the drug is present in the tissues and correspondingly little in plasma. V_d = 1.0 l/kg means that 4% of the drug is present in the plasma. A large V_d corresponds to a long half-life. The total amount of the drug present in the body can be calculated by multiplying the V_d by the concentration in plasma when the distribution has achieved an equilibrium.

Steady state refers to the condition (with long-term medication) where the amount of the drug administered per time unit is equal to the amount eliminated per time unit. If the dosage interval is shorter than the half-life, the concentration in serum will gradually increase with repeated administration until the patient reaches a steady state, as shown in Fig. 23.

A steady state is achieved with first-order kinetics because an increase in the amount administered leads to increased elimination. Drugs with a half-life of a few hours rapidly achieve a steady state because so

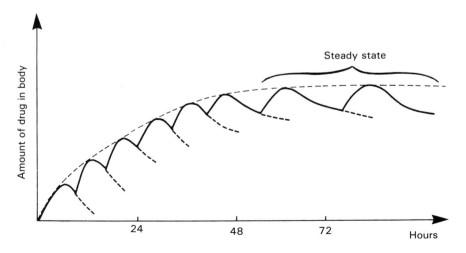

FIGURE 23. Dosage of a drug to the point where a steady state is achieved.

much is excreted during the interval between doses. Drugs with a long half-life take longer to achieve a steady state with a therapeutic concentration in serum because such small amounts are metabolized in the intervals between doses. The noneliminated remainder accumulates in the body. A steady-state concentration at a therapeutic level can be achieved more rapidly if the drug is given in larger, "loading" doses. A good rule of thumb is that a steady state can be achieved after four to five half-lives unless loading doses are given.

During maintenance treatment the best effect is obtained if the intervals between doses correspond roughly to the biological half-life. This gives a more level concentration in serum and avoids accumulation.

Clearance (CL). Clearance can be defined as

$$\text{Clearance} = \frac{\text{rate of elimination}}{\text{concentration of drug}}$$

In first-order kinetics the rate of elimination increases in proportion to the concentration of the drug. Clearance of such drugs is therefore constant within the range of drug concentrations in clinical use, and the term does not indicate how much of the drug is being eliminated, but rather the volume of plasma that is completely free of it.

The relationship between half-life, volume of distribution, and clearance is given by the equation

$$T_{1/2} = 0.693 \times \frac{V_d}{CL}$$

5

Peripherally Acting Analgesics and Glucocorticosteroids

PERIPHERALLY ACTING ANALGESICS

These drugs inhibit pain chiefly in areas peripheral to the central nervous system, that is, at the nociceptors (pain receptors) in the tissues. Recent evidence suggests, however, that some of the drugs also have an analgesic effect in the central nervous system. Most of them inhibit prostaglandin synthesis, which partly explains their mechanism of action. The prostaglandins (PGs) are formed from phospholipids (lipids with a polar head group and a fatty acid backbone) in the cell membrane (see Fig. 24). Phospholipase A_2 (a phospholipid-cleaving enzyme) cuts off arachidonic acid, which is an unsaturated fatty acid with 20 carbon atoms, from the phospholipids. This cleavage takes place continuously at a low rate but is greatly increased by physical, chemical, or hormonal stimuli, as in tissue injury. The cells contain two different enzymes, cyclooxygenase and lipoxygenase, that are both able to act on arachidonic acid. Cyclooxygenase converts arachidonic acid to a cyclic endoperoxide known as PGG_2. The PGG_2 has a very short half-life and is transformed into PGH_2 plus a free oxygen radical. This oxygen radical is very highly reactive and probably contributes to the activation of pain receptors. PGH_2 can be converted to the prostaglandins PGE_2 and $PGF_2\alpha$ and also to thromboxane A_2 and prostacyclin (prostaglandin I_2, PGI_2). The type of prostaglandin or leukotriene produced depends on the type of cell and on the external stimulus.

The enzyme cyclooxygenase is inhibited by most peripherally acting

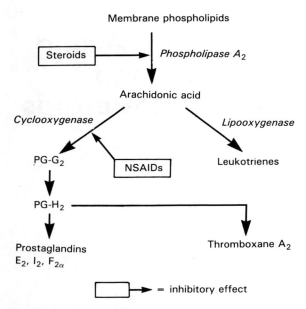

FIGURE 24. Effect of drugs on prostaglandin synthesis.

analgesics. The conversion of arachidonic acid by the enzyme lipoxygenase leads to the formation of leukotrienes, which are potent mediators in the inflammatory process. The ratio between prostaglandins and leukotrienes can influence the strength of the inflammatory reaction. PGE_2 is usually vasodilatory, while $PGF_2\alpha$ and PGI_2 can contract other smooth muscles. Thromboxane A_2, which is produced in blood platelets, increases their tendency to aggregate, while prostacyclin, which is produced in uninjured endothelium, inhibits the clotting of blood platelets.

As mentioned in Chapter 1, PGE_2 and PGI_2 make the nociceptors more sensitive to stimulation, which lowers the pain threshold. There is also evidence that PGE_2 contributes to the osteolysis seen in skeletal metastasis. Increased amounts of PGE_2 are probably produced in other forms of metastasis as well.

PGE_2 helps to maintain the efficiency of the mucosal barrier of the stomach, preventing the formation of gastric ulcers. The kidneys produce prostaglandins in order to maintain their blood supply under stress (decreased blood volume, hypertension, renal deficiency).

NONSTEROIDAL ANTI-INFLAMMATORY DRUGS (NSAIDs, ASPIRINLIKE DRUGS)

Although this group contains a number of drugs with qualitatively similar effects and side effects, there are important differences between them, and their effects are subject to great individual variations. (See Table 3.)

All the drugs in this group inhibit prostaglandin synthesis, most of them by competitive inhibition of cyclooxygenase. Aspirin inhibits this enzyme irreversibly; that is, the enzyme is destroyed and has to be synthesized again before new prostaglandins can be formed. Acetaminophen and diflunisal may act by scavenging the oxygen radicals formed during the synthesis of endoperoxides (see Fig. 24). This can lead secondarily to somewhat reduced prostaglandin synthesis and to inhibition of the anti-inflammatory effect of the endoperoxides. Diflunisal also directly inhibits the enzyme cyclooxygenase, and in high doses cyclooxygenase inhibitors lipooxygenase as well.

Analgesic and Anti-Inflammatory Properties

These drugs appear to have their analgesic effect through the inhibition of prostaglandin synthesis. Pain relief is usually obtained with lower doses than are required for an anti-inflammatory effect. At analgesic doses most of the prostaglandin synthesis is inhibited, so that it is doubtful whether the anti-inflammatory effect is due to the inhibition of cyclooxygenase, and the exact mechanism of the anti-inflammatory effect is not known. All these drugs are able to relieve pain and could theoretically be used as analgesics. This also applies to their use in rheumatic diseases, where the analgesic effect is probably very important clinically. Ordinary doses prob-

TABLE 3. Effect of Prostaglandins and Nonsteroidal Anti-Inflammatory Drugs (NSAIDs)

Effect on	Prostaglandin	NSAIDs
Nociceptors	Sensitization (lowered pain threshold)	Pain relief
Inflammation	Vasodilation	Anti-inflammatory[a] (at higher doses than for pain relief).
	Inhibition of polymorphonuclear granulocytes	Inhibition of polymorphonuclear granulocytes
Stomach	Strengthens mucous barrier	Increases tendency toward duodenal and gastric ulcer, owing to local erosion and probably systematic inhibition of prostaglandin synthesis
Hemostasis	Increases platelet adhesion (thromboxane A_2)	Prolongs bleeding time
Kidneys	Increases blood supply in response to stress (circulatory or renal insufficiency)	Can provoke edema and renal insufficiency

[a]Inhibition of prostaglandin synthesis (cyclooxygenase inhibition) without inhibition of leukotriene synthesis (lipoxygenase) can give rise to a strong inflammatory reaction. This is probably why some asthmatics become worse if they take an NSAID.

ably have less effect on inflammatory processes than on pain. However, the analgesic effect has a "ceiling." Doses above this level can have a greater anti-inflammatory effect but also a higher frequency of side effects. Some drugs seem to have a greater effect on pain than on inflammation, others less so. The reason for this is not known. There are also great individual variations.

Many of these drugs are slightly acidic and thus bind strongly to plasma proteins. During the inflammatory process the plasma proteins are released into the inflamed tissue, where, because of the acidity, the drugs no longer bind to the plasma proteins and are able to act therapeutically on the tissue. If the tissue has a low pH these drugs are less ionized and enter the cells by nonionic diffusion.

Antipyretic (Fever-Reducing) Properties

These prostaglandin synthesis inhibitors pass to some extent through the blood-brain barrier and have an antipyretic action, possibly by inhibiting the effect of prostaglandins on temperature regulation. Drugs like diflunisal, of which only a small proportion passes the blood-brain barrier, have a weaker antipyretic effect.

Effects on the Gastrointestinal Tract

The prostaglandins seem to play an important role in maintaining the resistance to acid of the mucous membrane of the stomach. They strengthen the mucous barrier, especially PGE_2. Inhibition of prostaglandin synthesis may therefore increase the sensitivity of the gastric mucosa to acid, which can lead to ulcer formation. Most NSAIDs also have a more or less localized erosive effect on the mucosa.

These drugs can give rise to abdominal pain and rarely to constipation or diarrhea.

Effect on the Kidneys

Prostaglandins are usually produced in the kidneys in small amounts. A reduced renal blood supply, however, will considerably increase the production of prostaglandins, whose vasodilatory action augments the blood supply. Patients with high blood pressure, edema, or slight renal insufficiency always have a high production of prostaglandins. If such patients receive prostaglandin synthesis inhibitors they may develop a moderate renal insufficiency with a tendency to fluid retention and edema. These drugs can also cause more serious renal failure.

Effect on Platelets and Granulocytes

Thromboxane A_2 increases the ability of platelets to aggregate. Thus, inhibition of thromboxane synthesis will reduce the aggregating capacity of the platelets and prolong the bleeding time. Prostacyclin (PGI_2), which is synthesized in the vessel walls, can to some extent counteract this effect, but since thromboxane synthesis is inhibited by lower concentrations of aspirinlike drugs than prostacyclin synthesis, the net effect is usually a tendency to increased bleeding.

Cases of aplastic anemia have been shown to occur in connection with virtually all NSAIDs, but only some pyrazolone derivatives (phenyl-butazone and oxyphenbutazone) have caused so many as to have clinical relevance.

Pulmonary Effects

About 10% of all asthmatics develop severe bronchoconstriction after taking NSAIDs. This is probably because the inhibition of cyclooxygenase increases the amount of arachidonic acid available for lipoxygenase, which converts it to leukotrienes, which can give rise to bronchoconstriction. Since all aspirinlike drugs have this property, a patient who reacts with an asthma attack to one drug will almost certainly have the same reaction to the others.

Effect on the Central Nervous System

A number of prostaglandins are also produced in the central nervous system, but their functions are not known exactly. They seem to be associated with temperature regulation and nausea, but not much is known about this. Aspirinlike drugs usually have few effects on the central nervous system, but some drugs (like indomethacin) often give side effects like headache, tiredness, and occasionally hallucinations.

Thus, in principle, all NSAIDs have qualitatively the same effects on the systems mentioned above. A great many new drugs in this group have appeared during the last few years; they are not always more effective than the older ones but may have fewer side effects.

ASPIRIN

Aspirin has been available as a painkiller since 1899 and is still one of the most frequently used analgesics. It has been used as a basis for the synthesis of a large number of analgesics, yet it was not until a few years ago that related drugs giving stronger pain relief were discovered.

Aspirin has analgesic, antipyretic, and anti-inflammatory properties. Its binding to cyclooxygenase is irreversible (i.e., it destroys the enzyme), in contrast to the other peripherally acting analgesics, which have a reversible binding to cyclooxygenase. Most of the effects of aspirin in the body are mediated by its main metabolite, salicylic acid. The drug does not inhibit prostaglandin formation in vitro but may do so in vivo. Whether or how this is related to the mechanism of action is not known.

Pharmacokinetics

The rate of absorption depends on the form in which it is administered. Solutions are most rapidly absorbed: usually 50% of the preparation is absorbed within 30 minutes. Enterosoluble and coated tablets are more slowly absorbed. They cause less local irritation in the stomach and are therefore more suitable for long-term use.

Aspirin is converted very rapidly (within 15 minutes) to salicylic acid, which has the same analgesic effect. The half-life of salicylic acid is 3 to 4 hours, and the action lasts about 4 hours, sometimes longer.

In the liver, salicylic acid is converted to metabolites that are excreted by the kidneys. A certain amount is also excreted in an unconverted form. One of the metabolites, gentisic acid, is strongly anti-inflammatory. Salicylic acid is eliminated according to first-order kinetics, but the enzyme capacity of the liver is exceeded by doses of more than 1–1.5 g of aspirin, and it is then excreted according to zero-order kinetics. The half-life is then increased to about 20 hours. At high doses (>6 g/24 hours) there is a risk of accumulation, with toxic effects. Constant use increases the enzyme capacity, which can be doubled. Salicylic acid is excreted in much greater quantities in alkaline urine.

Indications

Mild to moderate pain, especially from skeletal, muscular, and connective tissue. It is not really correct to describe aspirin and related drugs as "mild analgesics." When the dosage and indications are correct (as in pain with an inflammatory component), they can be more effective than the so-called strong analgesics.

Side Effects

Aspirin should not be used in any condition involving an increased bleeding tendency. Because aspirin binds irreversibly to and thus destroys cyclooxygenase, platelet aggregation is inhibited throughout the life of the platelets, about 8 days. A single does of aspirin therefore causes a prolonged bleeding time for about 4 to 7 days. These drugs must not be used in cases of esophageal varicose veins or peptic ulcer. About 10% of all asthmatics react to aspirin with bronchoconstriction and prolonged asthma attacks. In such cases all inhibitors of prostaglandin synthesis are contraindicated.

Dosage

The dosage is 0.5–1.0 g four to six times a day. The analgesic effect does not increase with doses over 1 g, but the anti-inflammatory effect does. Tinnitus and dizziness are signs of overdose.

DIFLUNISAL

Diflunisal is a fairly new drug, a difluorophenyl derivative of salicylic acid, but with quite different pharmacological properties. Diflunisal seems to inactivate oxygen radicals and has a certain directly inhibiting effect on cyclooxygenase. The analgesic effect lasts for 8–12 hours and is usually stronger than that of aspirin or acetaminophen. In some studies of acute pain the analgesic effect has been found to be at least as strong as that of acetaminophen plus codeine. Diflunisal has been tested on cancer patients in pain and has been found to have a definite effect on pain from skeletal and soft-tissue tumors. Like the other NSAIDs, it has both analgesic and anti-inflammatory properties, but it has very little antipyretic effect, since most of it does not pass through the blood-brain barrier.

Pharmacokinetics

The half-life is dose dependent. At doses of 500 mg twice a day the half-life is 10–12 hours, and it decreases with decreasing doses. Maximum pain relief is obtained after 3 to 4 hours. Diflunisal is excreted in the form of glucuronide conjugates in the urine.

Side Effects

Diflunisal has a less negative effect on the gastrointestinal tract than aspirin and in the therapeutic doses it has little effect on blood platelets.

Dosage

The dosage is 250–500 mg twice a day. If a rapid effect is required an initial dose of 1000 mg can be given.

ACETAMINOPHEN

Acetaminophen has an analgesic and antipyretic effect equivalent to that of aspirin for most types of pain. It is less effective for pain of rheumatic origin, however, and is therefore not used as an anti-inflammatory drug. Studies of edema formation after tooth extraction have shown that acetaminophen may inhibit edema formation better than aspirin does, which indicates that it may have an anti-inflammatory effect, at any rate at an early stage of the process, and especially in inflammation due to trauma. It is not known exactly how acetaminophen acts, but it does not appear to have much effect on prostaglandin synthesis, although it may inhibit cerebral cyclooxygenase. Acetaminophen acts as a free-radical scavenger, and this may partly explain why it reduces certain types of inflammation. In rheumatic diseases the tissues contain large numbers of granulocytes and other cells that produce free oxygen radicals. The capacity of acetaminophen to scavenge these is greatly exceeded, so that it has little anti-inflammatory effect in rheumatic diseases. But it must be emphasized that there is much we do not know about the mechanism of action of acetaminophen.

Pharmacokinetics

Acetaminophen is completely absorbed and usually reaches its maximum effect within 2 hours. The half-life is 2 hours, and the effect lasts for 4 to 5 hours.

Acetaminophen is metabolized in the liver to inactive metabolites that are conjugated and excreted in the urine. During degradation in the liver toxic intermediary products are formed and rapidly inactivated by the glutathione system. If the capacity of this enzyme system is exceeded the toxic intermediary products accumulate and bind covalently to cell proteins. This causes cell necrosis.

Recent findings have shown that acetaminophen may have a carcinogenic effect if given in massive doses to rats or mice for 6 months to a year. These doses, however, are so high that they induce liver cell necrosis, which has been shown to have an unspecific carcinogenic effect in several systems. The doses are many times the size of ordinary therapeutic doses, and no signs of carcinogenic effects have been found at normal doses.

Indications

Mild to moderate pain.

Side Effects

Therapeutic doses seldom give rise to side effects. Acetaminophen has little effect on the hemostatic system and has no ulcerogenic effect on the gastric mucosa. It provokes no cross-allergic reactions with salicylates and can be safely given to asthmatics.

Overdosage produces liver cell necrosis, which can arise after 10–15 g. Twenty-five grams can be fatal if the intoxication is not treated within 10 hours with methionine or N-acetylcysteine.

Dosage

The recommended dosage is 0.5–1.0 g three to five times a day. Usually a dose of 1 g is necessary to obtain a satisfactory effect.

INDOLE DERIVATIVES: INDOMETHACIN AND SULINDAC

Indomethacin has good anti-inflammatory and analgesic properties.

Pharmacokinetics

The half-life is 4 to 7 hours. The drug is metabolized in the liver to inactive metabolites and is excreted mainly as glucuronides in the urine and to some extent in the feces.

Side Effects

Unfortunately, up to 50% of patients have side effects with daily doses of 75 mg or more: 1–3% have hallucinations, 25–50% have headaches, and a good many have gastrointestinal complaints. This drug seems to have more side effects than newer NSAIDs, but it has been known and used for many years and is very well tolerated by many patients.

Dosage

The recommended dosage is 50–200 mg a day in three to four doses.

Sulindac is structurally very similar to indomethacin but the clinical effects are quite different. It is a prodrug. This means that it has to be absorbed in the gastrointestinal tract and converted to active substances in the liver in order to act as an analgesic, anti-inflammatory, or antipyretic agent. It thus seems to have fewer gastrointestinal side effects than the other drugs in this category because it has little direct effect on the gastric mucosa. It is a good analgesic and is well tolerated.

Pharmacokinetics

Sulindac has a half-life of 8 hours, while the active sulfide metabolite has one of 16 hours, so it can be administered twice a day.

Indications

Pains in the musculoskeletal system and soft tissue.

Side Effects

Sulindac has fewer gastrointestinal side effects than aspirin and has little effect on renal function.

Dosage

The recommended dosage is 200 mg in the morning and evening.

PROPIONIC ACID DERIVATIVES: NAPROXEN, IBUPROFEN, KETOPROFEN, FENOPROFEN, FLURBIPROFEN, AND FENBUFEN

These drugs probably have less pronounced anti-inflammatory effects than high doses of indomethacin and aspirin, but they have fewer side effects and are better tolerated. Both the anti-inflammatory effect and the side effects are dose dependent. Many of the published reports on NSAIDs showing differences between the various drugs really show differences in dose levels.

Pharmacokinetics

The half-lives of naproxen and fenbufen are 10–17 hours, and they can thus be given morning and evening. The half-lives of ketoprofen, ibuprofen, flurbiprofen, and fenoprofen are 2 to 5 hours, and they must be given three to four times a day for continuous pain relief. Being quickly absorbed and rapidly reaching a steady state, the four latter drugs are very suitable for fluctuating pain.

Indications

The propionic acid derivatives are indicated in cases of pain from the musculoskeletal system and soft tissue. The analgesic effect is at least as good as that of aspirin and in some studies has been shown to be as good as that of a combination of aspirin and codeine.

Dosage

Naproxen and fenbufen, 250–500 mg morning and evening; fenoprofen and ibuprofen, 200–600 mg three to four times a day; flurbiprofen and ketoprofen, 50–100 mg two to three times a day.

OXICAM DERIVATIVE: PIROXICAM

Piroxicam is an oxicam derivative that resembles propionic acid derivatives as regards effects and side effects.

Pharmacokinetics

The drug has a half-life of 36–45 hours and one dose a day is therefore sufficient. It takes 5 to 7 days to achieve a steady state. Drugs with a long half-life need to be used with caution in cancer patients, however, since these patients become easily dehydrated and the cancer may alter the functioning of liver and kidneys. Such drugs can then have long-lasting toxic effects.

Indications

Pain in the musculoskeletal system and soft tissue.

Dosage

The recommended dosage is 10–30 mg once a day.

PYRAZOLONE DERIVATIVES: PHENYLBUTAZONE, ANTIPYRINE, AND AZAPROPAZONE (APAZONE)

Phenylbutazone is a highly effective anti-inflammatory and analgesic agent. However, its use is limited by the serious side effects such as aplastic anemia and agranulocytosis. It also fairly often gives rise to edema. Antipyrine and azapropazone are much less toxic and are probably also less effective than phenylbutazone.

Pharmacokinetics

Phenylbutazone has a half-life of 50–100 hours, while antipyrine and azapropazone have half-lives of 4–7 and 10–15 hours, respectively.

Indications

Musculoskeletal pain.

Dosage

Phenylbutazone, 200–600 mg daily in two to three doses; azapropazone, 300 mg daily in three to four doses; antipyrine, 500–1000 mg daily in three to five doses.

GLUCOCORTICOSTEROIDS

This group of drugs has immunosuppressive and anti-inflammatory properties. Salts and fluids are retained to a varying extent (mineral corticoid effect; see Table 4). The drugs act particularly on the early vascular phase in the inflammatory response, inhibiting the formation of edema and the migration granulocytes and lymphocytes and also the functions of these cells, causing the release of fewer lysosomal enzymes, lymphokines, and so forth. They therefore also have a pain-relieving effect, which takes place within hours to days. The slow onset of action is probably due to the fact that corticosteroids interact with DNA to induce synthesis of specific proteins, such as lipocortins, which inhibit phospholipase A_2 and reduce the synthesis of prostaglandins and leukotrienes (see Fig. 24).

TABLE 4. Comparison of Glucocorticosteroids

	Equivalent anti-inflammatory dose (mg)	Gluco-corticosteroid effect	Mineral corticosteroid effect	Biological duration of action (hours)
Cortisone	25	0.8	0.8	8–12
Hydrocortisone	20	1.0	1.0	8–12
Prednisolone	5	4.0	0.8	15–50
Prednisone	5	3.5	0.8	15–50
Triamcinolone	4	5.0	0	15–50
Dexamethasone	0.75	25.0	0	36–72
Betamethasone	0.50	25.0	0	36–72

SIDE EFFECTS

The side effects depend on the dosage and length of treatment. Doses corresponding to 15–20 mg of prednisone per day usually give few side effects even over a long period.

Musculoskeletal System and Soft Tissue

Glucocorticosteroids inhibit the production of vitamin D and probably the formation of osteoblasts. This results in an increased incidence of osteoporosis, but this usually affects only risk groups such as postmenopausal women and elderly people generally. High doses given over a long period can give rise to myopathy, with proximal muscular atrophy.

Endocrine System

Patients with a reduced capacity for insulin secretion can develop hyperglycemia. This may be followed by diabetes, which can rapidly develop into ketoacidosis.

Glucocorticosteroids have a negative feedback effect on ACTH, resulting in the suppression of endogenous cortisol production. After a while this will cause atrophy of the adrenal cortex, leading to suppression of the production of sex hormones. This situation can be exploited in the treatment of sex hormone-sensitive tumors.

Gastrointestinal Tract

Glucocorticosteroids increase the risk of developing a peptic ulcer, and caution should be exercised with patients with a history of ulcer or bleeding disturbances. At doses of less than 20 mg prednisolone per day, however, the risk is slight.

Psychological Side Effects

These side effects vary from euphoria to dysphoria and depression. Regular psychosis rarely occurs. Usually, however, these drugs have a mentally stimulating effect.

Risk of Infection

Steroid therapy increases the risk of developing an infection and often masks a nascent infection. But in the doses recommended for palliative treatment in the later stages of cancer this problem is rare.

USE OF GLUCOCORTICOSTEROIDS
FOR THE RELIEF OF SYMPTOMS
IN CANCER PATIENTS

Treatment of Pain

Because of their ability to counteract inflammation and reduce edema, steroids can relieve pain from skeletal metastases, compression of nerves and blood/lymph vessels, stretching of the organ capsule (e.g., in liver tumors), intra-abdominal tumors, tumors in the pelvis, soft-tissue tumors, and intracranial tumors. They also have a directly analgesic action, apart from their anti-inflammatory action, possibly through their inhibition of prostaglandin synthesis.

By suppressing the production of sex hormones by the adrenal cortex, exogenously administered glucocorticosteroids can relieve pain in hormone-sensitive cancers of the prostate and breast, especially if the gonads have been removed or irradiated.

Hypercalcemia

Some patients with metastases develop hypercalcemia, which is manifested by symptoms such as diffuse pain, anorexia, nausea and vomiting, psychological symptoms, and a generally poor state of health. Steroids can reduce such hypercalcemia (see Chapter 7).

Anorexia and Cachexia

Glucocorticosteroids can increase the appetite and improve the general health of these patients, sometimes with startling effects. A patient who is emaciated may appreciate the common side effects of increased weight and facial fattening.

Palliative treatment with recommended doses seldom gives other side effects. Autopsies of over 500 patients with terminal cancer showed that the only risk involved in glucocorticosteroid therapy was an increase in the incidence of peptic ulcer with complications. Death due to bleeding or perforation occurred in 5% of steroid-treated patients, as opposed to 1% of untreated ones.

6

Centrally Acting Analgesics

Centrally acting analgesics all bind to opioid receptors in the central nervous system and relieve pain by increasing the activity in some of the endogenous pain-inhibiting systems. This means that they bind to receptors in the dorsal horn of the spinal cord on both the primary afferent nociceptive neurons and the nociceptive spinothalamic tract neurons. They also increase activity in the descending pathways from the periaqueductal gray matter and the rostral ventral medulla (see Fig. 11). In addition, they influence limbic structures and thus the emotional components of the pain experience. Morphinelike analgesics do not alter the pain threshold, but they reduce the pain and increase tolerance to it. Spinal, polysynaptic reflexes are also diminished. The various drugs differ pharmacokinetically and pharmacodynamically—that is, with regard to their effects at the receptor level.

PHARMACODYNAMICS

We do not know exactly how a chemical substance provokes a physiological response via a receptor on the cell membrane. The effect can be measured quantitatively, however, by administering increasing amounts of the substance being tested and expressing the results as a dose-response curve, as shown in Fig. 25.

The substance represented by the left curve in the figure has the highest activity per molar unit. In other words, it is the most potent. Both

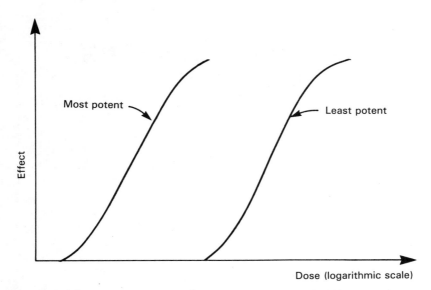

FIGURE 25. Dose-response curves for two pure agonists with different potencies.

substances, however, have the same maximum effect, so in the appropriate doses they are equally effective in clinical use.

Definitions of Pharmacodynamic Terms:

Agonist: substance that binds to a receptor and has a physiological effect.
Antagonist: substance that binds to a receptor without producing a physiological effect and that can counteract the effect of an agonist.
Partial agonist: substance that binds to a receptor and produces a physiological response with a maximum effect that is less than that of a pure agonist (see Fig. 26). In other words, a partial agonist has a weaker intrinsic effect than a pure agonist.
Affinity: an expression of the ability of a drug to interact with ("bind to") a receptor. The affinity does not correlate with the maximum effect. The various centrally acting analgesics have different affinities to the appropriate opioid receptors and different intrinsic effects.

OPIOID RECEPTORS

Morphinelike analgesics and endogenous opioids bind to several types of receptors, but with different affinities. An overview of the different effects obtained by stimulation of the different receptors is given in Table 5.

Binding to the various receptors is not entirely selective. Morphine, for example, will also bind to kappa, sigma, and delta receptors, but to a much lesser extent than to mu receptors.

Binding to the mu receptors is thought to explain the effect of mor-

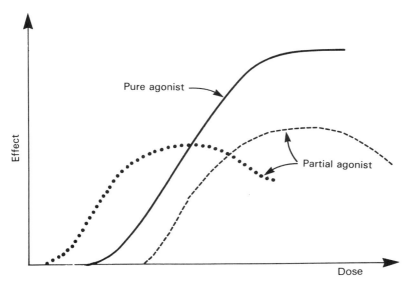

•••••• Partial agonist with higher affinity than a pure agonist
------- Partial agonist with lower affinity than a pure agonist

FIGURE 26. Dose-response curves for pure and partial agonists.

phine. Recent research indicates that there may be two types of mu receptors, mu_1 and mu_2. Stimulation of mu_1 is thought to produce analgesia without depressing respiration, a finding that could have good therapeutic results if it could be exploited in the development of new drugs.

Depending on the physiological response produced by the binding

TABLE 5. Probable Effects of Opioid Receptors

Receptor	Effects	Pure or partial agonists
Mu_1	Analgesia (mainly supraspinal), physical dependence (similar to morphine), hypothermia (high doses), antidiuretic effect, miosis	Morphine, methadone, beta-endorphin, buprenorphine
Mu_2	Respiratory depression, bradycardia (high doses), gastrointestinal motility	
Kappa	Analgesia (in spinal medulla), sedation, no respiratory depression, physical dependence similar to nalorphine	Nalorphine, pentazocine, dynorphin
Sigma[a]	Physical effects: dysphoria, feeling of unreality, hallucinations, nightmares	Nalorphine, pentazocine
Delta	Analgesia	Enkephalins
Epsilon	Unknown	Beta-endorphin

[a]Functionally but not morphologically defined.

to the receptor, opioids are classified as pure agonists, partial agonists, mixed agonists/antagonists, and pure antagonists. Pure agonists are capable of producing the maximum biological response. Partial agonists (buprenorphine) have a weaker intrinsic effect and cannot produce the maximum biological response (see Fig. 26). This means that there is a limit to the analgesic effect, and higher than recommended doses can cause an increase in the drug's antagonistic properties, resulting in a decrease in pain relief and an increase in side effects.

If a drug with a higher affinity for opioid receptors than morphine is given together with morphine in normal doses, the two drugs will have an additive effect because there will be enough receptors available for both of them. In very high combined doses, however, all the receptors will be occupied, and the drug with the higher affinity (e.g., buprenorphine) will prevail over morphine at the receptor level. It may then act antagonistically to morphine. This is seldom a problem in clinical practice, but if a patient has been taking high doses of morphine over a long period, treatment with buprenorphine may increase the pain and at worst give rise to abstinence symptoms.

EFFECTS OF OPIOIDS

Analgesia

Opioids are usually classified as strong or weak (see Table 6). At high doses the side effects can prevent analgesia. This applies to codeine, propoxyphene, and meperidine (in chronic dosage). Morphine can be administered in very high doses without the side effects increasing more than the analgesic effect. The mechanism of action of the partial agonists and the antagonists means that doses above a certain level can cause diminishing analgesia. The clinical consequences of this are that although these drugs act as strong analgesics in acute pain, in certain cases they are un-

TABLE 6. Classification of Centrally Acting Analgesics (Opioids)

	Agonists	Partial agonists/antagonists
Weak	Codeine Oxycodone Propoxyphene	Pentazocine (per os)
Strong	Morphine Methadone Meperidine Hydromorphone Levorphanol Heroin	Buprenorphine Pentazocine (parenteral) Nalbuphine Butorphanol

TABLE 7. Effect of Opioids on Different Types of Pain

Type of pain	Effect
Deep-seated, aching, somatic or visceral	Very good
Bone pain	Some effect
Pain on activity/movement	
Nerve compression	
Decubitus	
Muscle spasms	Variable, often inadequate
Colic/tenesmus	
Burning, superficial pain	Usually no analgesic effect,
Postherpetic neuralgia	only sedative
Dysesthesia/allodynia	

suitable for the treatment of severe chronic cancer pain, because a cancer patient may need much higher doses than are necessary to relieve acute pain. (see Table 7.)

Respiratory Depression

All opioids reduce the sensitivity of the respiratory center to carbon dioxide, which under physiological conditions is the main stimulator of respiration.

Pain stimulates the respiratory center and thus counteracts the inhibiting effect of opioids.

When strong analgesics are given in doses that satisfy a cancer patient's requirements for chronic pain relief, the accompanying respiratory depression has no practical significance even if normal doses are considerably exceeded. The increasing tolerance to the analgesic effect is reflected in a corresponding increase in tolerance to the respiratory depression.

Combinations of opioids with other drugs that depress the central nervous system should be used with caution, however, especially during the first phase of the treatment.

Sedation

Most patients become drowsy at the beginning of opioid therapy. When the pain diminishes the patient is able to relax and make up for all the sleep lost during nights of pain. Opioids also have a directly sedative effect and a correct dosage causes drowsiness for the first few days.

After 3 to 5 days of regular dosing, the drowsiness diminishes and most patients have adequate pain relief without feeling disturbingly sedated.

Confusion and Hallucinations

These side effects are most common in debilitated and elderly patients. They may be a sign of overdosage, but they also occur with correct doses.

Dizziness and Unsteadiness

These symptoms also occur most often in elderly patients and may be due to postural hypotension or to a disturbance of the vestibular system.

Euphoria and Risk of Psychological Dependence

The emergence of drug addiction as a widespread problem during the last three decades has meant that this side effect of opioid drugs has attracted a lot of interest and has led to a great reduction in the use of opioids even when they are medically indicated. However, a number of studies have indicated that when morphine is used for the relief of cancer pain it does not lead to abuse. Correctly administered, opioids are not psychologically addictive. Cancer patients are not primarily interested in getting high, but in becoming free of pain.

Depression

Some patients develop symptoms of depression after long-term therapy with opioids. This may be caused by an aggravation of the disease, which in itself is depressing. Opioids may cause depression, however, and some patients need to take antidepressants to control the symptoms.

Development of Tolerance

Tolerance is usually used to mean that the effect of a drug diminishes with prolonged use. A better definition in the case of strong analgesics is that the dose needs to be increased over time in order to maintain the analgesic effect. The development of tolerance is a normal biochemical process in the chronic use of strong analgesics, so that many people worry that morphine-type drugs will lose their power to relieve pain after a time. In practice, however, the dose can be increased to obtain the same effect, so there is no need to wait until a patient has reached the terminal stage before administering opioids in order to maintain the effect until death. In fact, the opposite course gives better results: if treatment is started at an early stage the patient is more likely to experience adequate pain relief during all phases of the disease.

Tolerance develops to all the effects of morphine, but it develops at different speeds. Tolerance to the sedative effect and often to accompanying nausea develops rapidly, but that to analgesia and respiratory depression takes longer. Tolerance to miosis and constipation develops very slowly. This means that a patient can easily become constipated even with doses that are suboptimal for pain relief.

Tolerance develops much more quickly with intramuscular and even more so with intravenous administration than with oral administration. The latter is therefore a preferable method in cases of chronic pain. Tolerance usually develops most rapidly during the first and second months of treatment, after which it is often not necessary to alter the dose for a long time.

If an unusually rapid increase in dosage is required, this may indicate that the patient has a type of pain that responds only partly to opioid analgesics. It may also be due to the influence of psychological, social, or religious factors on the patient's experience of the pain, and these should be taken up with the patient and dealt with as far as possible. Another reason may be that the pain is increasing because the disease is worsening.

In some patients the dosage can be reduced toward the terminal stage, but there are great individual variations, depending on the development of the disease.

Centrally acting analgesics must not be withdrawn suddenly. If a patient has used one of these drugs for a fortnight or more, a sudden withdrawal will give symptoms of abstinence. Restlessness and anxiety may be followed by more pronounced signs, such as nasal and lacrimal secretion, rapid breathing, sweating, and dilated pupils. These signs may be followed by tachycardia, tremors, nausea and vomiting, and diarrhea.

Nausea and Vomiting

All opioids lead to nausea and vomiting in a certain number of patients. There are probably three underlying mechanisms:

1. Stimulation of dopaminergic neurons in the chemoreceptor trigger zone for emesis (CTZ) in the area postrema of the medulla.
2. Sensitization toward emetic impulses from the vestibular system.
3. Inhibition of peristalsis in the gastrointestinal tract, accompanied by a tendency toward gastric stasis and constipation.

Because the vestibular system is probably affected, the nausea is most pronounced in ambulant patients. No clear differences have been found between the various drugs, but the tolerance of an individual patient to the drugs may vary, so that pronounced nausea with methadone treatment may be relieved by changing to morphine, or vice versa.

Nausea and vomiting are usually worst at the start of the treatment and tend to decline gradually, since tolerance develops more rapidly than it does to the pain-relieving effect. Some patients, however, show no signs of nausea at first and only develop these symptoms after several days or weeks.

There is no definite relation between nausea and the size of the dose of a strong analgesic. Morphine has been claimed to have an emetic effect at relatively low doses, but at higher doses it can have an antiemetic effect. Pain can also cause nausea, and in such cases treatment with morphine may cause the nausea to diminish.

Effect on the Gastrointestinal Tract

Morphine and similar analgesics inhibit peristalsis in the gastrointestinal tract and cause increased contraction of the sphincters. This leads to delayed gastric emptying and consequently slows down the absorption of drugs. Morphine increase the pressure in the bile ducts, which can cause stomach pains. Almost everyone on long-term opioid therapy suffers from constipation. Morphine seems to be the most strongly constipating agent, while buprenorphine and pentazocine are less so. All patients on long-term therapy with strong analgesics should also be given laxatives.

Effect on the Urogenital System

Morphine has an antidiuretic effect, but this is not usually strong enough to have any clinical importance. Morphine increases the contraction of the sphincter of the urinary bladder, and urine retention can arise in predisposed people. This occasionally happens during epidural administration of morphine but is relatively rare with oral administration. Some patients develop urgency incontinence.

Release of Histamine

This effect of morphine is highly individual and occurs seldom. Some people react strongly, with peripheral vasodilation and hypotension; some develop bronchoconstriction and asthma. Patients who react to morphine in this way do not usually react to the other opioids with histamine release, but such drugs should still be administered with caution and preferably not intravenously or intramuscularly. Drugs with the least possible chemical resemblance to morphine should be chosen.

ORAL ADMINISTRATION OF OPIOIDS

All strong analgesics are absorbed from the small intestine but are metabolized to a varying extent during their first passage through the liver (first-pass metabolism), and only part of the administered dose reaches the target organs. This is why morphine was considered for a long time to be ineffective if administered orally. Their bioavailability when taken orally varies a great deal from patient to patient—equal doses of morphine can produce up to fivefold differences in plasma concentration in different patients (see Table 8). Opioids therefore have to be given in doses that are individually tailored according to the response, and standard dosages cannot be used. There is no definite relation between relief of pain and plasma concentration, so an analysis of the level in serum is of little clinical use.

Equianalgesic Doses

Table 9 shows equianalgesic doses for various preparations in this group. The reference analgesic is morphine, 10 mg administered parenterally. No equianalgesic effect can be obtained between high doses of morphine and meperidine (prolonged use), buprenorphine, or pentazocine.

PURE AGONISTS

MORPHINE

Morphine has a strong analgesic effect, unsurpassed by any of the other opioids. It has a purely agonistic effect by binding to the opioid receptors involved in pain relief (mostly mu receptors). Thus in theory there are no limits to the analgesic effect, but side effects may preclude the giving of high enough doses.

Pharmacokinetics

Morphine is easily absorbed from the small intestine, but the high first-pass metabolism gives it reduced bioavailability, since only 20–50% enters the systemic circulation. There are great individual differences here. Usually an oral dose needs to be two or three times as high as a parenteral dose, so if the oral doses are high enough, the results obtained may be as good as the results with injections.

Most of an administered dose of morphine is converted in the liver to glucuronic acid and excreted in the urine, but other metabolites are also formed. The active metabolite *morphine-6-glucuronide* is formed in such small quantities that it probably has very little analgesic effect, but in renal insufficiency it will not be effectively excreted. The serum concentration will then rise considerably and a strong analgesic effect may be produced, which may even result in intoxication. We do not know whether the other metabolites have any analgesic effect. Five to ten percent of a dose of morphine is excreted in unconverted form in the urine.

TABLE 8. Biological Availability of Orally Administered Opioids

Opioid	Approximate percentage
Morphine	35 ± 20
Heroin	35 ± 20
Methadone	80 ± 15
Levorphanol	ca. 50
Meperidine	35 ± 20
Hydromorphone	ca. 20
Codeine	ca. 70
Propoxyphene	ca. 20
Pentazocine	ca. 20

TABLE 9. Equianalgesic Doses and Duration of Action

Drug	Equianalgesic dose (parenteral administration) (mg)	Equianalgesic dose (oral administration) (mg)	Duration of action (hours)
Morphine	10	20–50	3–5
Heroin	5	15–40	3–5
Hydromorphone	1–2	5–15	3–5
Levorphanol	2	3–6	4–8 (chronic dosage)
Methadone	10	10–20	Single dose: 4 Chronic dosage: 8–12
Meperidine	100	300	2–4
Buprenorphine	0.3–0.6	0.4–0.8 (sublingually)	4–6
Pentazocine	45–60	Not attainable	2–3

The half-life of morphine is 2 to 4 hours and is not affected by chronic use, which means that a steady state is rapidly achieved. There is no danger of accumulation.

The effect lasts for about 4 hours, which means that it has to be administered every 4 hours around the clock to obtain chronic relief.

Slow-Release Morphine Tablets

One of the disadvantages of morphine is the short-lasting effect, and the recent manufacture of morphine in the form of slow-release tablets represents a great step forward. These are absorbed slowly from the intestine over a period of 6 to 8 hours, so that the effect lasts for 8 to 12 hours. The daily dose is the same as for liquid morphine, and most studies show that the effects and side effects are the same as for the liquid form. Some patients find that the nausea provoked by the oral solution ceases with these tablets. The tablets are also easy to administer in ambulant therapy.

Indications

Morphine is indicated for severe pain.

Dosage

For oral solution or conventional tablets, the ordinary initial dosage is 5–10 mg orally, usually 10 mg. Elderly patients should be given the lowest dose. If adequate relief has not been obtained after two to four doses, the dose can be increased by 50–100%, depending on the initial dose. If the effect is still not good, the dose should be increased until relief is obtained (see Chapter 10).

For morphine slow-release tablets, a good treatment regimen is to start with conventional tablets or oral solution and then, when the optimal dose has been found, to continue with the same daily dose in the form of slow-release tablets.

Side Effects

The different types of side effects have been described above under Effects of Opioids and will be discussed further in Chapter 10. Long experience with morphine has shown that it has relatively few subjective side effects and a good analgesic effect compared with other opioids in the treatment of chronic cancer pain.

HYDROMORPHONE

Hydromorphone is chemically related to morphine and has much the same effect. A dose of 1.5 mg intravenously is equianalgesic to 10 mg of morphine.

Pharmacokinetics

Hydromorphone is absorbed from the small intestine and probably has a bioavailability of 30–50% with considerable interindividual differences. Its half-life is 3 to 4 hours. It is slightly shorter-acting than morphine. Owing to its high solubility, it may be given intramuscularly in a solution (10 mg/ml) that is two to four times more concentrated than morphine on an equianalgesic basis.

Indications

Severe pain.

Side Effects

These are very similar to those of morphine.

HEROIN

Heroin is diacetylmorphine, a semisynthetic derivative. It is not presently available in the United States.

Pharmacokinetics

Heroin is readily absorbed in the intestine. It is fairly rapidly deacetylated to 6-acetylmorphine and morphine, the active metabolites. Heroin is more soluble than morphine, which is an advantage for injections in cachectic patients. It has a slightly more rapid onset action than morphine, and the duration of action is 3 to 5 hours.

Indications

Severe pain.

Side Effects

Heroin is more strongly sedative than morphine and causes slightly less vomiting.

CODEINE

Codeine comes from the opium poppy and is an intermediary product in the natural synthesis of morphine.

An analgesic effect can be obtained with 30 mg administered orally, and the analgesic effect of 60 mg orally corresponds to that of 300–600 mg of aspirin. For a long time it was thought that 5–15% of an administered dose of codeine was metabolized to morphine in the liver, which was thought largely to explain the analgesic effect. Recent studies, however, indicate that only about 3–5% is converted to morphine and that the most important effect comes from codeine per se.

Pharmacokinetics

Codeine is easily absorbed from the small intestine, and the bioavailability is 70–80% when it is administered orally. The half-life is 2 to 6 hours and is unaffected by chronic use. This means that chronic use of high doses does not involve a risk of accumulation. The effect lasts 3 to 4 hours. Eighty percent of the drug is metabolized in the liver, and the remainder is excreted unconverted in the urine.

Indications

Codeine is indicated for moderate pain and is used in conjunction with a peripherally acting analgesic. It is also indicated for cough and diarrhea.

Side Effects

Codeine can cause drowsiness. Nausea, vomiting, and dizziness are most frequent in ambulant patients. It can also cause constipation and over a long period the tolerance to the analgesic effect is greater than to the constipation, so that patients who use the same dose for a long time may find that the pain relief diminishes while the constipation remains. This applies to all other centrally acting analgesics. Predisposed patients can develop dyskinesia of the biliary tract.

OXYCODONE

Oxycodone is a derivative of codeine and has much the same properties.

Pharmacokinetics

Oxycodone is rapidly absorbed from the small intestine and has a bioavailability of 50%. The duration of action is 3 to 4 hours.

Indications

Moderate pain. It should be used in combination with aspirin or acetaminophen.

Dosage

Five to ten milligrams every 4 to 6 hours.

Side Effects

These are the same as for codeine.

MEPERIDINE

Meperidine is a synthetically manufactured analgesic, which arose out of an attempt to make a spasmolytic drug from atropine. This attempt was not successful, but it led to the accidental discovery that meperidine had a strongly pain-relieving effect, and meperidine has since been used as an analgesic.

Pharmacokinetics

Meperidine is chiefly administered parenterally. When given orally it has a high first-pass metabolism, and three times as much must be used in oral as in parenteral administration. Absorption from the rectum is slow and uncertain, and the analgesic effect is weaker than with injections.

Meperidine is metabolized in several ways, but the most important clinically is demethylation to normeperidine. Normeperidine has a considerably longer half-life than the parent drug, and when used chronically it accumulates. This metabolite causes side effects from the central nervous system in the form of tremors, agitation, and myoclonus and seizures. These effects are dose dependent and can occur in connection with chronic use in cancer patients (>300 mg orally per dose). Thus the side effects set an upper limit for the chronic use of meperidine as an analgesic, even though it is a pure agonist.

The half-life of meperidine is 2 to 5 hours. The duration of action is only 2 to 4 hours, so that it has to be taken more often than morphine.

Indications

Meperidine is indicated for moderate to severe pain.

Side Effects

Meperidine has a less spasmogenic effect on the gastrointestinal tract than morphine and may therefore be more suitable for use in colic. It causes more pronounced drowsiness than morphine and because of its relationship with atropine, it often makes the mouth feel very dry.

As mentioned above, chronic use of fairly high doses causes an accumulation of toxic metabolites, which leads among other things to tremors and sometimes myoclonus and seizures.

Dosage

The equianalgesic dose, which has the same analgesic effect as 10 mg of morphine administered parenterally, is 100 mg. An oral dose of 300 mg is required to obtain the same effect. It must be given every 2 to 4 hours for continuous pain relief.

METHADONE

Methadone is also a synthetic strong opioid. Its chemical structure is closely related to that of propoxyphene.

Pharmacokinetics

Methadone has a better bioavailability after oral intake than any of the other opioids, and 65–90% of the drug enters the systemic circulation after passing through the liver.

Methadone is distributed in the body according to the two-compartment model. In other words, it has two half-lives, one in the alpha phase (corresponding to the central chamber) lasting 2 to 5 hours, and one in the beta phase lasting 22 to 59 hours. The situation after one dose is shown in Fig. 27.

After one dose methadone will relieve pain for about 4 hours. If further doses are given at intervals of 4 to 6 hours, the drug will gradually have a prolonged effect, since it accumulates because of the long half-life in the beta phase. The plasma concentration will now remain at a therapeutic level for a long time because elimination in the steady state is chiefly dependent on the half-life in the peripheral compartment, as shown in Fig. 28.

Methadone therefore possesses the great advantage that it needs to be administered only two to four times a day once it has reached a steady state. This can give a patient a whole night's sleep without pain.

If the drug continues to be administered every 4 hours, it can accumulate in the body and give symptoms of intoxication (Fig. 29). It is metabolized in the liver and excreted in the urine. The pH value of the urine has a great influence on the half-life (in the beta phase), which is about 20 hours if the urine is acidic and can be over 40 hours if the urine is alkaline.

Side Effects

Methadone causes less contraction of the gastrointestinal sphincters than morphine. The most dangerous side effects arise from accumulation in the

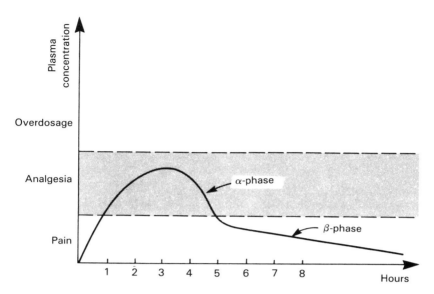

FIGURE 27. Concentration of methadone in serum after a single dose.

body caused by excessively large and/or frequent doses. One of the first signs of intoxication is increasing sedation. Methadone may cause hallucinations more frequently than morphine. It needs to be used with great caution by elderly people, since they may have a reduced metabolism and eliminate the drug more slowly.

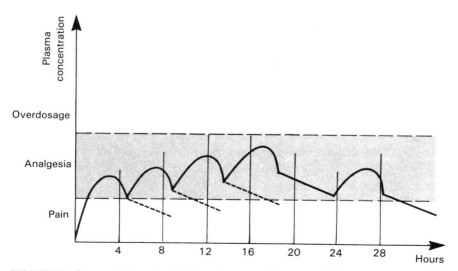

FIGURE 28. Concentration of methadone in serum after repeated doses.

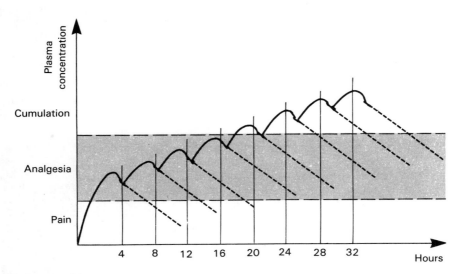

FIGURE 29. Concentration of methadone in serum after doses every 4 hours.

Dosage

The equianalgesic dose is 10 mg administered parenterally. Since it has a strong tendency to irritate the tissues, it is not very suitable for parenteral therapy.

It is obvious from its pharmacokinetic properties that methadone must be given frequently at first. Later, it usually needs to be taken only two to four times a day.

The usual initial dose is 5–10 mg orally, five or six times a day for 1 to 3 days. After this it is usually given every 8 hours. The usual dose is 20–40 mg per day, but this can vary from 10 mg to over 100 mg. (A more practical description of how to establish the dosage is given in Chapter 10.)

PROPOXYPHENE

The chemical properties of propoxyphene are closely related to those of methadone, and the pharmacokinetics and mechanism of action are similar. The analgesic effect of propoxyphene, however, is weaker.

The analgesic effect is similar to that of codeine, but, like methadone, propoxyphene needs to be administered in successive doses to obtain the maximum effect, unless a loading dose is given first. Thus, 65 mg of propoxyphene chloride has about the same analgesic effect as 0.5 g of aspirin. This corresponds to about 30 mg of codeine in one-dose studies. In multiple-dose studies 45–60 mg of codeine is usually required to approximate the effect of 65 mg of propoxyphene chloride.

Pharmacokinetics

Propoxyphene is easily absorbed from the small intestine, but 60–80% is broken down during the first passage through the liver. Distribution takes place according to a multicompartment model. The half-lives are 3 to 4 hours in the alpha phase and about 12 hours in the beta phase. It should therefore not be given more often than three to four times a day. The drug is metabolized in the liver to norpropoxyphene, which has a half-life of 29–43 hours. Long-term administration of fairly high concentrations can therefore lead to a high concentration of this metabolite, which in high doses has an effect similar to that of lidocaine and can cause mental disturbances, heart arrhythmia, and convulsions.

Indications

Propoxyphene is indicated for moderate pain and should be used in combination with a peripherally acting analgesic.

Side Effects

These consist of drowsiness, nausea and vomiting, and constipation, but propoxyphene is less constipating than codeine.

Toxicity

A single dose of ten to twenty 70-mg tablets of propoxyphene combined with alcohol can be fatal. The symptoms of overdose are depressed respiration, sometimes respiratory arrest, convulsions, heart arrhythmia, and lung edema.

Dosage

Propoxyphene chloride should be given 70–140 mg two to four times a day, and propoxyphene napsylate 100–200 mg two to four times a day.

PARTIAL AGONISTS AND MIXED AGONISTS-ANTAGONISTS

Nalorphine is an antidote to morphine. It has a high affinity to opioid receptors but little analgesic effect. It has slightly agonistic properties (a partial agonist) and strongly antagonistic properties. It has strong mental side effects.

PENTAZOCINE

Pentazocine is a development of nalorphine. It is an agonist for kappa and sigma receptors and an antagonist for mu receptors. It is thus a mixed agonist and antagonist, but in therapeutic concentrations the agonistic properties predominate. When the dose is increased above the therapeutic level the analgesic effect does not increase correspondingly (see Fig. 26), but the side effects do, and this prevents overdosing.

Pharmacokinetics

Pentazocine is absorbed fairly slowly after intramuscular injection, and the peak plasma concentration is reached after 1 to 2 hours. When it is injected intravenously, the peak effect is obtained after 15–60 minutes. When taken orally, the drug is slow-acting. It has a low bioavailability when administered in tablet form or in an oral solution. Only 15–30% is unchanged after the first passage through the liver.

The half-life is 2 to 3 hours and the effect lasts about the same time. The drug is metabolized in the liver and excreted through the kidneys as glucuronides.

Indications

Parenterally administered, pentazocine is indicated for moderate to severe pain. In cases of mild to moderate pain it can be given orally. It should be taken together with a peripherally acting analgesic.

Side Effects

Psychotomimetic side effects are experienced by 5–30% of patients after therapeutic doses and are most frequent in connection with high doses. The drug can cause hallucinations, strange feelings, nightmares, and disorientation. This is particularly difficult for cancer patients, who may be feeling emotionally unstable anyway. These side effects can be explained by the fact that pentazocine has a great affinity for the sigma receptor.

In higher therapeutic concentrations pentazocine has a negative effect on the blood circulation by causing peripheral vasoconstriction and having a negative inotropic effect on the heart. Great care must therefore be taken if the drug is given intravenously to patients with cardiac insufficiency.

Pentazocine has little constipating effect and does not cause histamine release. When given subcutaneously or intramuscularly, it fairly often gives rise to subcutaneous infiltrates and occasionally gives rise to muscular necrosis. It can also cause nausea, vomiting, and dizziness.

Dosage

The parenteral equianalgesic dose is 45–60 mg. The recommended oral dose (25–50 mg) has an analgesic effect corresponding to approximately 0.5 g of aspirin. Clinical studies have shown that with oral therapy the drug does not effectively relieve severe pain because the side effects preclude high enough doses. The drug must be given every 3 hours for chronic pain. Oral doses of 25–100 mg can be given for moderate pain, preferably together with a peripherally acting analgesic. The only advantage of pentazocine over codeine and propoxyphene is that it is less constipating.

BUPRENORPHINE

Buprenorphine is a semisynthetic strong analgesic. Structurally it resembles morphine, and it is a partial agonist for the mu receptor. This means that the analgesic effect has a ceiling—if the dose is increased beyond the point where the maximum effect is obtained, there is a risk that the analgesic effect will diminish (see Fig. 26).

Pharmacokinetics

The drug can be administered only by injection or in the form of sublingual tablets. It begins to take effect within 15–30% minutes irrespective of the method of administration. With sublingual tablets the maximum effect is obtained after 1 to 2 hours. Buprenorphine has a high affinity for the mu receptor, and the analgesic effect therefore lasts longer than the plasma concentration would indicate. Thus the effect lasts 4 to 8 hours even though the half-life in plasma is only about 3 hours. The drug is more potent and has a weaker intrinsic effect than morphine, which means that the maximum effect is less.

Buprenorphine is metabolized in the liver. The breakdown products are excreted mainly through the bile and feces, but about one-third are excreted in the urine.

Chronic use does not cause accumulation in the body.

Indications

Buprenorphine is indicated for moderate to severe pain.

Side Effects

These are qualitatively the same as those of morphine, but the negative effect on the gastrointestinal tract is small, and there is little constipation. The drug is more of a sedative than morphine. Nausea and vomiting are more common than with morphine treatment, but there are individual differences, so that some patients tolerate it better than morphine.

Buprenorphine causes the same degree of respiratory depression as morphine. Because of the strong receptor affinity the depression is not entirely reversed by naloxone, and after an overdose the respiration-stimulating drug doxapram must be used as well.

Buprenorphine has no negative effect on the circulation and, in contrast to pentazocine, it has no pronounced psychotomimetic side effects.

Dosage

The equianalgesic dose is 0.3–0.6 mg administered parenterally. Somewhat higher doses can be given if necessary. The maximum single dose is thought to be 1.2 mg. As with the other opioids, tolerance develops to buprenorphine, but usually this cannot be entirely compensated by an increase in the dose.

In patients who have taken morphine over a long period, the transition to buprenorphine can give rise to abstinence symptoms and increased pain because of buprenorphine's partially antagonistic properties. With ordinary therapeutic doses, however, the transition from morphine to buprenorphine is normally uncomplicated.

WHICH OPIOIDS SHOULD BE CHOSEN TO TREAT CHRONIC PAIN IN CANCER PATIENTS?

COMBINATIONS WITH PERIPHERALLY ACTING ANALGESICS

Codeine, propoxyphene, and pentazocine should be combined with peripherally acting analgesics. Used alone, their analgesic effect is no stronger than that of the peripherally acting drugs, and they usually have more side effects. The point of the combination is to create an additive analgesic effect by having two different mechanisms of action (peripheral and central), while keeping the side effects down to an acceptable level.

These combinations should satisfy the following requirements:

1. They should not have more than two components.
2. The components should have different mechanisms of action.
3. Each component should be present in a dose that would have an analgesic effect when used alone. This means that the following minimum amounts should be used:

Aspirin	500 mg
Diflunisal	250 mg
Acetaminophen	500 mg
Ibuprofen	200 mg
Fenoprofen	200 mg
Naproxen	250 mg
Fenbufen	250 mg
Flurbiprofen	50 mg
Ketoprofen	50 mg
Indomethacin	25 mg
Piroxicam	20 mg
Codeine	30 mg
Propoxyphene chloride	65 mg
Propoxyphene napsylate	100 mg
Pentazocine	25–50 mg

Many compound drugs contain too small a dose of one or more of the active constituents, so that care should be taken to select the right compound.

4. The components should have approximately the same pharmacokinetic properties and the same duration of action.

The advantage of *fixed combinations*—that is, both constituents in the same tablet—is that they are easy to use and reduce the number of pills the patient has to take. Acetaminophen or aspirin combined with codeine satisfies all four of the above requirements. Propoxyphene has a much longer half-life than the two peripherally acting drugs mentioned above, so if the doses are given often enough for the peripherally acting constituent to have a continuous effect, this can lead to accumulation of the centrally acting constituent at higher doses. Propoxyphene is thus best combined with diflunisal, naproxen, or some other long-acting peripheral analgesic.

Tolerance does not develop to the peripherally acting constituent, but it does of course to the centrally acting one. This means that over a long period the centrally acting component will start to lose some of its analgesic effect. The side effects (especially constipation) usually remain for a long time.

Free combinations—that is, where the centrally and the peripherally acting components are in separate tablets—have the advantage that the dose of centrally acting analgesic can be increased without altering the dose of the other component, so that the pain relief is qualitatively better.

STRONG CENTRALLY ACTING ANALGESICS

Meperidine and pentazocine are not suitable for the treatment of chronic cancer pain. Meperidine has a more short-lasting effect than morphine and its use in fairly high doses over a long period leads to accumulation of toxic metabolites, which affects the central nervous system. The drug also leads to dry mouth. Pentazocine is effective for only 2 to 3 hours and has unpleasant side effects at high doses. It is not effective against severe pain when given orally. Nalbuphine and butorphanol are not available for oral use and therefore not suitable for long-term treatment.

Methadone and morphine are effective for oral treatment of severe pain. These drugs are pure agonists, with no ceiling for the analgesic effect, so that the dose can be increased until the desired effect is achieved.

Methadone has the advantage of a long-lasting effect and consequently needs to be taken less often. It provides relief for a whole night at a time. It is particularly suitable for ambulant patients whose general condition is fairly good and who have fairly stable pain. A certain amount of training is required to administer the correct dosage and avoid accumulation. Levorphanol is an alternative to methadone but has a somewhat shorter duration of action.

Morphine has to be given every 4 hours in oral solution or tablet form. In the form of slow-release tablets, however, the effect lasts 8–12 hours. Its advantage over methadone is that it has a long-lasting effect without the risk of accumulation. Thus it is easier to administer to patients in poor general health than methadone because there is less risk of over-dosing. Morphine in oral solution or conventional tablets is very suitable for fluctuating pain because the short half-life means that a steady state is achieved quite quickly. An alternative to oral morphine is hydro-morphone.

Morphine, heroin, and hydromorphone are all equally effective for parenteral use at the terminal stage, but heroin and hydromorphone are available in high-potency injectable form for cachectic patients. The solubility of morphine (40 mg/ml) is sufficient for the vast majority of patients. All three drugs can be given every 4 hours or more often if necessary. Methadone is less suitable, since the injections cause local irritation, especially if they are intravenous. Only morphine, hydromorphone, heroin, or buprenorphine should be used for continuous subcutaneous infusion with a drug delivery pump, since the other drugs cause local irritation.

Clinical experience with buprenorphine administered as sublingual tablets or intramuscularly for cancer pain indicates that the effect is similar over a short period but that buprenorphine has rather more side effects. Over a longer period many patients stop using buprenorphine, and in most cases it has to be replaced by morphine or methadone.

Generally speaking, there seems to be a lot of confusion among health professionals about the different effects and side effects of the various opioids. Many of them are afraid to give patients morphine because they think it is more dangerous than meperidine or hydromorphone. There are no rational grounds for thinking this. Most health professionals are happy to give pentazocine, even though from the patients point of view this drug is the least satisfactory choice for severe pain. In general, one can say that these drugs are often given in insufficient doses at too long intervals.

7

Psychotropic Drugs

ANTIDEPRESSANTS

Antidepressants can be divided into four groups according to their chemical structure and supposed mechanism of action: tricyclic antidepressants, monoamine oxidase (MAO) inhibitors, atypical antidepressants, and tetracyclic antidepressants. The tricyclic antidepressants can be subdivided into tertiary and secondary groups, depending on whether there are three or two methyl (CH_3) groups bound to the nitrogen in the side chain (Fig. 30).

MECHANISM OF ACTION

The mechanism of action of antidepressants is still fairly obscure. Ninety percent of the transmitter substances norepinephrine and serotonin released into the synaptic cleft are reabsorbed by the presynaptic neuron. The tricyclic antidepressants prevent liberated transmitter substances from being taken up again, so that the concentration in the synaptic cleft increases (see Fig. 31). This is traditionally held to increase transmission in the serotonergic and noradrenergic pathways, which counteracts depression. It is thought that tertiary tricyclic antidepressants mainly influence the serotonin synapses, while the secondary tricyclic antidepressants increase transmission in the nerve pathways where norepinephrine is the neurotransmitter.

Tertiary tricyclic antidepressants

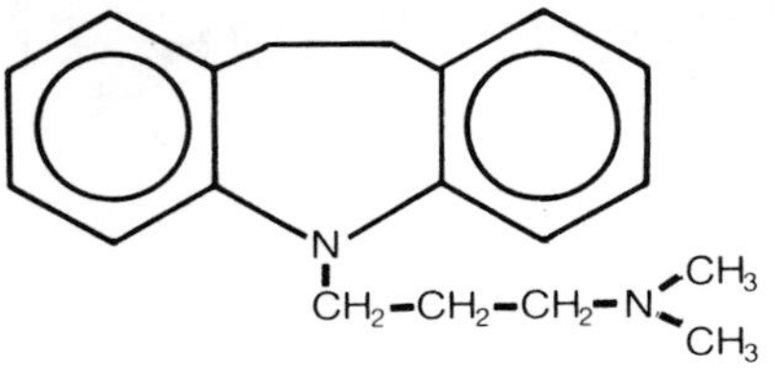

Secondary tricyclic antidepressants

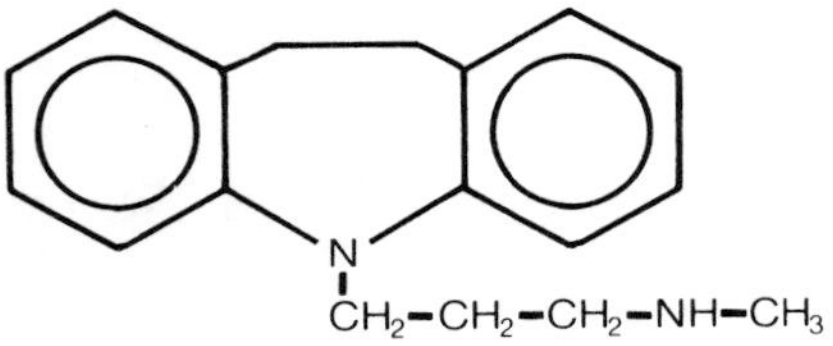

Tetracyclic antidepressants

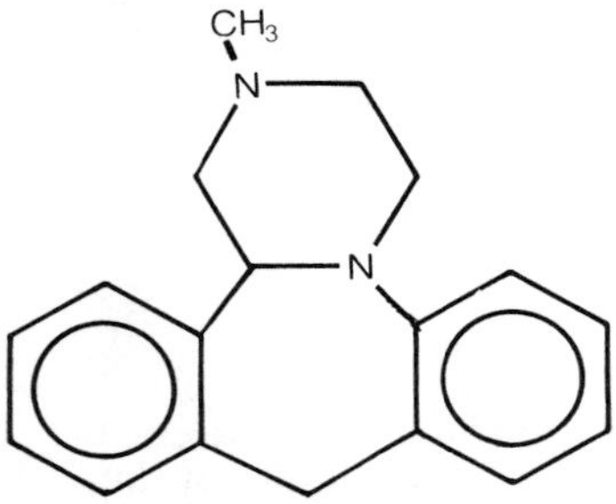

FIGURE 30. Chemical structures of antidepressants.

As the name indicates, MAO inhibitors decrease the degradation of transmitter substances, which results in an increased pool of biogenic amines. Whether this effect is clinically important, however, has not been established.

Atypical antidepressants like trazodone are thought to be relatively specific inhibitors of the reuptake of serotonin, but they almost certainly have other, so far unknown, mechanisms of action.

The mechanism of action of the tetracyclic antidepressants is even less clear than that of the tricyclic ones. Situated on the presynaptic membrane is an alpha$_2$ receptor to which liberated norepinephrine binds, and this binding may give a negative feedback. Mianserin probably blocks this alpha$_2$ receptor, leading to an increased turnover of norepinephrine. The effect on serotonergic synapses is still less clear. Mianserin also blocks H$_1$ and H$_2$ histaminergic receptors.

The side chain in the tricyclic antidepressants has a certain structural similarity to acetylcholine, and these drugs therefore have a fairly high affinity for cholinergic receptors. They have almost no intrinsic effect, so that their antagonistic properties are dominant, and they have anticholinergic (side) effects. Mianserin and trazodone have no such side chain and therefore lack affinity for cholinergic receptors. This means that anticholinergic symptoms are minimal with these drugs. They are no more effective as antidepressants than the tricyclic antidepressants but are preferable in cases where the latter give rise to anticholinergic side effects or where the patient is taking other drugs with anticholinergic side effects.

The endogenous pain-inhibiting mechanisms involve both serotonergic and noradrenergic neurons, and clinical trials have shown that the tertiary tricyclic antidepressants can increase tolerance to pain. Antidepressants act on the central nervous system at several levels and also have a favorable effect on the limbic system. In animal experiments antidepressants have been shown to potentiate the endogenous pain-inhibiting

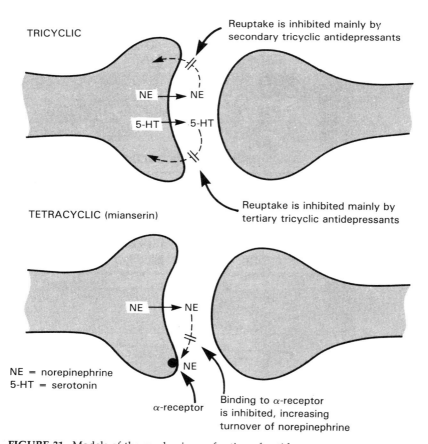

FIGURE 31. Models of the mechanisms of action of antidepressants.

mechanisms and analgesics, but this relation has not been established for clinical nociceptive pain syndromes.

Tricyclic antidepressants (especially amitriptyline) are useful in the treatment of neurogenic, superficial, burning pain (dysesthesia). The effect is unrelated to the antidepressive effect, since the pain is usually relieved within 1 to 5 days and usually at lower doses than those used for antidepressive therapy. It has been claimed that amitriptyline counteracts dysesthesia by blocking peripheral receptors in the nerves, possibly the muscarinergic, cholinergic, $alpha_1$-adrenergic, and H_1 or H_2 histaminergic receptors.

The anxiety-relieving effect of tricyclic antidepressants begins within 1/2 hour to 2 hours. The release of inhibitions and the motor stimulation become noticeable after 3 to 10 days, while the real antidepressive effect (psychostimulatory, a lightening of mood) usually has a latency time of 1 to 5 weeks.

Relief from anxiety is usually obtained after a week with mianserin, and the other effects generally occur after the same intervals as with the tricyclic antidepressants.

PHARMACOKINETICS

Tricyclic Antidepressants

Absorption from the gastrointestinal tract is good. There is high first-pass metabolism, since the tertiary amine drugs are to some extent demethylated to secondary amine drugs. The first-pass metabolism is very individual, however, and a given dose can produce very different plasma levels. The dosage therefore needs to be adjusted according to the patient's reaction. If there is no clinical effect an analysis of the plasma concentration may be indicated. The drugs have high plasma protein binding and a large apparent distribution volume (V_d), and the half-life is 12–20 hours.

Some tricyclic antidepressants (nortriptyline, chlorimipramine) have a clinical effect only within a limited range of concentrations, and here the correct dosage is essential (see Fig. 32).

Tetracyclic Antidepressants

Mianserin is rapidly absorbed and the peak plasma concentration is achieved within 1 to 3 hours. It is metabolized in the liver to less active metabolites. Seventy percent is excreted in the urine and the rest in the feces. The half-life is on average 17 hours but can vary from 6 to 39 hours.

Atypical Antidepressants

Trazodone is well absorbed after oral administration, and if taken shortly after the ingestion of food it may be absorbed in larger amounts. It has a biphasic elimination with a half-life of 3 to 6 hours in the initial phase and a terminal half-life of 5 to 9 hours, with relatively large interindividual variations.

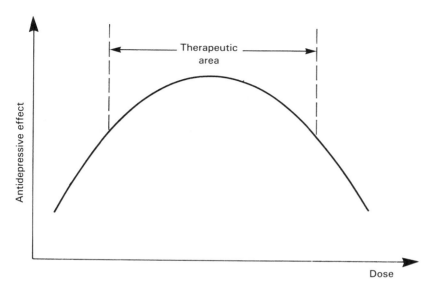

FIGURE 32. Dose-response curve of nortriptyline.

SIDE EFFECTS

The most pronounced side effects are the anticholinergic ones, including dryness of the mouth, tachycardia, urine retention in predisposed individuals, increased ocular pressure in those with narrow-angle glaucoma, and accommodation paresis. Postural hypotension and even heart failure can occur with high doses and where there is predisposing heart disease. All these effects are less pronounced with mianserin and trazodone. The sedative effect is different for each drug, as shown in Table 10.

TABLE 10. Classification of Antidepressants

	Anxiety relief	Sedative	Anticholinergic
Tertiary tricyclic			
Amitriptyline	+ + +	+ + +	+ + +
Doxepin	+ + +	+ + +	+ +
Imipramine	+ +	+ +	+ +
Chlorimipramine	+ (+)	+ (+)	+ (+)
Trimipramine	+ + (+)	+ + +	+ +
Tetracyclic			
Mianserin	+ + [a]	+ + +	−

[a]Latency period, 3–7 days.

DOSAGE

Antidepressive Therapy

Tricyclic Antidepressants

The treatment should be started with relatively small doses: 10–25 mg two to three times a day. After this the dosage should be gradually increased over 3–10 days until it reaches 150–225 mg one to three times a day. The dosage should be regulated according to the side effects and the clinical effect. Elderly patients may be very sensitive to these drugs, and very low doses should be used at first.

Other Antidepressants

A dose of 30 mg mianserin in the evening should be given the first week; after this it can be increased to 60–90 mg or even higher doses. The starting dose of trazodone is 100 mg/day in more than one dose, increasing to 200–400 mg/day.

With all these groups of drugs, the dosage should be reduced to the lowest possible maintenance dosage for 3 to 6 months once the clinical effect has been obtained.

Antianxiety Therapy

Tricyclic Antidepressants

The dosage is 25–75 mg a day in one or more doses.

Tetracyclic Antidepressants

The dosage is 30–60 mg in the evening.

Hypnotic Therapy

Tricyclic Antidepressants

The dosage is 10–75 mg doxepin, amitriptyline, or trimipramine 1 to 2 hours before bedtime.

Tetracyclic Antidepressants

The dosage is 30–60 mg in the evening, 2 hours before bedtime.

Pain Relief

High doses of an antidepressant can combine well with a peripherally acting analgesic. If used with an opioid, the dose of antidepressant often needs to be reduced because of the additive sedative effect. The ordinary dosage of a tricyclic antidepressant in combination with an opioid is 10–25 mg two to three times a day, or 10–75 mg in the evening. The use of mianserin, trazodone, or MAO inhibitors on these indications is so far very limited. Elderly or very debilitated patients may be extremely sensitive to antidepressants and may become confused.

Dosage of 25–75 mg a day of a tricyclic antidepressant is usually sufficient to treat neuropathic pain.

NEUROLEPTICS

These drugs, which have been shown to be very useful in the treatment of psychotic patients, have also been discovered to alleviate a number of other symptoms. Their clinical effect is probably due to the blocking of various receptors.

1. The blocking of *dopamine receptors* has an antipsychotic effect and also extrapyramidal side effects, such as symptoms resembling Parkinsonism. The dopamine receptor block also produces an antiemetic effect.
2. The blocking of *alpha-adrenergic receptors* produces peripheral vasodilation and a tendency to hypotension and hypothermia.
3. The blocking of *muscarine receptors* ("acetylcholine receptors") has peripheral anticholinergic effects. Centrally, the extrapyramidal effects of the dopamine receptor block are inhibited, because the balance between the cholinergic and dopaminergic motor pathways is reinstated. The blocking of this receptor in the central nervous system produces sedation.
4. The neuroleptic syndrome is produced by unknown mechanisms and consists of psychomotor inhibition without loss of intellectual functions.

Neuroleptics can be roughly divided into low-potency and high-potency drugs, as shown in Table 11. There are many of these drugs on the market, and it is beyond the scope of this book to describe each one in detail.

LOW-POTENCY NEUROLEPTICS

Low-potency neuroleptics (see Table 11) act on all the above-mentioned types of receptors. They thus have a stronger unspecific sedative hypnotic effect than those in the high-potency group. The side effects are primarily due to the effects on the autonomic nervous system (anticholinergic action) and the cardiovascular system, resulting in hypotension, among other things. In elderly people such drugs can lead to a reduced blood supply to the brain and a state of confusion.

Chlorpromazine in doses of 10–25 mg two to three times a day can

TABLE 11. Classification of Neuroleptics

Low-potency neuroleptics
  Propylamino-phenothiazines
    Chlorpromazine
    Methotrimeprazine
    Promazine
    Chlorprotixene
    Tioridazine
High-potency neuroleptics
  Piperazine-phenothiazines
    Dixyrazine
    Perphenazine
    Prochlorperazine
  Butyrophenone derivatives
    Haloperidol

suppress anxiety and restlessness. The drug has not been shown conclusively to potentiate the analgesic effect of opioids. Some patients react with dysphoria.

Methotrimeprazine seems to potentiate the analgesic effect of opioids and in high concentrations has an analgesic effect of its own. It is a strong norepinephrine-blocking agent but has a less marked effect on dopamine and acetylcholine receptors. Methotrimeprazine has a side chain like that of trimipramine and a strongly sedative and hypnotic effect, which may be an advantage in the treatment of pain at night, but which limits the use of the drug during the day. The dosage is 5–25 mg one to three times a day.

HIGH-POTENCY NEUROLEPTICS

High-potency neuroleptics are more specifically antagonistic to dopamine and have less effect on the other receptors. They therefore have a less unspecific sedative effect and few anticholinergic and cardiovascular side effects. The extrapyramidal side effects are more common, although they seldom occur with doses in the range usually used for treating cancer patients. These drugs have a stronger specifically suppressive effect, calming emotional tension and causing reduced spontaneous activity and greater indifference to external stimuli, including pain. They are good antiemetics.

Perphenazine and prochlorperazine are equally good for treating anxiety and nausea in cancer patients. Their action is slightly sedative. The dosage is 5–10 mg two to four times a day.

Haloperidol is even less sedative and may even have a slightly stimulating effect. Doses of 0.5–2.0 mg one to three times a day are often sufficient.

Flupentixol in small doses calms anxiety and may counteract depression and stabilize mood. It may have a stimulating and elevating effect and should therefore be given early in the day. A more strongly sedative drug may need to be given in the evening. The dosage is 0.5–1.0 two to three times a day, usually in the morning and afternoon.

TRANQUILIZERS AND HYPNOTICS

The use of these drugs for cancer patients is no different from their use in other clinical situations and will not be dealt with in any detail here.

The benzodiazepines are very good antianxiety agents. When taken during the day they are usually not strongly sedative, even though they are effective hypnotics. The benzodiazepines should generally be used cautiously because they tend to be addictive, but this cannot be considered a problem as regards cancer patients with a poor prognosis. They usually do not potentiate the effect of analgesics on somatic pain, but they may relieve certain types of neuropathic pain, probably because the patient is more relaxed and therefore secretes less epinephrine and norepinephrine, which can trigger pain in such conditions.

Many of these drugs, such as diazepam and chlorazepate (Tranxene), have long half-lives (20–80 hours), and they are broken down to active metabolites that sometimes have even longer half-lives. This means that there is a risk of accumulation with long-term use. Oxazepam (Serax) and lorazepam (Ativan), which have half-lives of 8–20 hours and are converted to inactive metabolites, are therefore suitable for patients with reduced liver function (e.g., liver metastasis).

Meprobamate, promethazine, and the barbiturates may occasionally have an excitatory and antianalgesic effect. This should be remembered when deciding which antianxiety or hypnotic drug to use.

Antidepressants and neuroleptics are useful drugs for treating anxiety and insomnia in cancer patients suffering from pain.

Hydroxyzine differs from the other tranquilizers in that it has been shown in some studies to potentiate the analgesic action of morphine. Hydroxyzine is an antihistaminic drug with calming and antiemetic properties, which also helps to reduce itching. It is thus useful for cancer patients with pain and nausea.

USE OF PSYCHOTROPIC DRUGS IN CANCER PATIENTS WITH PAIN AND OTHER DISTRESSING SYMPTOMS

ANALGESIC EFFECT

Analgesics are generally the best drugs for treating pain and they should be used as far as possible. If they do not seem to have a satisfactory effect, the dose should be increased. Merely augmenting the analgesic effect is not usually good indication for using a neuroleptic or antidepressant, which ought to be given for the sake of their other properties. Studies have shown, however, that some neuroleptics and/or antidepressants can increase the analgesic effect of opioids in the treatment of pain, and hydroxyzine has been found to add to the action of strong analgesics. Methotrimeprazine and hydroxyzine can also have an analgesic effect on their own, and some tricyclic antidepressants, such as amitriptyline, can relieve neuropathic pain (dysesthesia) in many patients.

RELIEF OF OTHER SYMPTOMS

Nausea and vomiting. These symptoms may be caused by the disease itself or by opioids or other drugs. Neuroleptics can relieve the nausea and enable the patient to continue taking the opioid and thus obtain adequate pain relief (see Chapter 11, p. 163).

Confusion and hallucinations are not unusual in connection with the use of opioids. Confusion is dose dependent and ceases when the dose is reduced, but this of course may cause the pain to return. Hallucinations are usually not dose dependent, and in such cases a different centrally acting analgesic can be tried. If this does not help, a potent neuroleptic may allow high doses of an analgesic to be given without the recurrence of hallucinations or confusion.

Sedation/apathy. Opioids have a sedative effect at first, but this declines after about 3 to 7 days. Some patients do remain sedated, although this may be due to the disease.

The first pain-killing mixtures (Brompton cocktail) contained cocaine to counteract the sedative effect and increase pain relief, but the cocaine had a number of psychiatric side effects (e.g., hallucinations, insomnia, and reduced appetite) and did not increase the analgesia, so the combination was discontinued. Apathetic patients may occasionally be stimulated by cocaine, and here the recommended dose is 5–20 mg four times a day, with the largest doses given early in the day. This is used very rarely.

Depression, anxiety, and insomnia. Low-potency neuroleptics can cause depression, and more potent neuroleptics, such as butyrophenones, are safer from this point of view. Psychotropic drugs should be given in lower doses, especially at first, to patients taking opioids than to others, mainly because opioids also have a sedative and antianxiety effect and the two types of drugs can strongly potentiate each other.

8

Nerve Blocks, Neurosurgery, and Nerve Stimulation

NERVE BLOCKS

The aim of nerve blocks is to block the pain impulses before they reach the spinal cord. Sometimes nerve blocks can be used *diagnostically* to establish where the pain is coming from. For example, the blocking of certain somatic nerves can confirm or refute that a pain originates from the area supplied by the nerves, although in practice it can be difficult to obtain an unambiguous answer.

Prognostic block: Here local anesthetics are used to test the possible effect of a permanent block. Only if the local anesthetic is effective can a destructive permanent block be considered.

Therapeutic block: A local anesthetic or neurolytic agent is used to achieve an effect that may last for weeks or months. Ideally only the pain impulses are supposed to be blocked, but in nerves that transmit both sensory and motor impulses, both will naturally be affected. The most common ways to destroy the nerve fibers (neurolysis) are by means of ethanol, 50–96%; phenol, 5–7% in aqueous solution; or phenol, 5–10% in glycerol as a hyperbaric fluid. Therapeutic blocks are divided into blocks of the somatic nervous system and blocks of the autonomic, sympathetic nervous system.

A nerve block should be considered when a cancer patient's pain stems from one or very few areas and when the pain is so severe that it cannot be controlled by moderately strong analgesics in adequate doses. A successful block will prevent or at any rate delay the use of strong opioids. Blocks are most effective when they are carried out at a fairly early stage, and the effect may be less good if the patient has been using opioids for some time. Long-term use of opioids is not, however, a reason for not trying a nerve block.

After a neurolytic block the injured nerves will begin to regenerate, which may cause distressing neuropathic pain, especially in somatic nerve fibers. Neurolytic blocks are therefore usually carried out only on patients who are thought to have less than a year to live. Neurolytic blocks are very seldom given to patients with a normal life expectancy, except for sympathetic nerve blocks (block of the celiac plexus or the lumbar sympathetic trunk).

SOMATIC NERVE BLOCKS

Local Infiltration in a Lesion

Many cancer patients suffer from pain in the musculoskeletal system. The pain may be caused by increased muscular tension due to anxiety, compensatory spasms in the muscles due to pain in other tissues, or inaction due to lying in bed. Localized, very tender infiltrates, known as myofascial trigger points, are often formed in the muscles. The pain from these can often be removed by injections of a local anesthetic, sometimes combined with a corticosteroid, but the effect does not last long and the treatment usually has to be repeated several times before a long-lasting effect is attained. The patient should also be offered additional treatment, for example, physiotherapy, if this is practicable.

Local injection of a local anesthetic combined with a corticosteroid in the region of superficial skeletal and soft-tissue metastases usually relieves the pain. Neuropathic pain due to peripheral nerve lesions with neuroma formation or scar shrinkage constricting a nerve can be relieved for short or long periods by injection of a local anesthetic with or without a corticosteroid in the painful area.

Blocking of Peripheral Nerves

The peripheral nerves are of several kinds and a neurolytic block will cause sensory and motor deficits. Another risk is that the block can result in a neuralgia that may be as severe as the original pain.

Intercostal/paravertebral block can be tried as a remedy in cases of localized tumor infiltration in the wall of the thorax or abdomen.

Block of the brachial plexus. Nerve blocks of the brachial plexus are often ineffective because movements of the arm, head, and neck produce traction of the nerves, which starts new pain impulses in spite of the block. A block can, however, provide relief from pain at rest. The advantages of a block must be weighed against the possibility of paresis of the arm.

Subarachnoid Block

To achieve a subarachnoid block, phenol in glycerol (a hyperbaric fluid) is injected into the subarachnoid space, and the patient is tilted in such a way that the liquid runs down and surrounds the afferent sensory dorsal roots at the level that is to be blocked. If done properly, this technique can achieve a fairly selective destruction of the sense of pain and temperature. It is often followed by a slight motor paresis, but this lasts only about 2 to 4 days. Occasionally it results in paraplegia, caused by thrombosis in the anterior spinal artery and the radicular arteries.

This type of block is indicated where the patient has a fairly well-defined area of pain, for example, pain in a leg or infiltration in the pelvic wall. A successful block will keep the patient free of pain for several months, and the block can be repeated several times if necessary.

This method has been less used in recent years since the introduction of epidural morphine administration, because the latter method is usually effective and has fewer side effects than subarachnoid neurolysis. For certain types of pain, however, the phenol block is preferable.

Epidural Block and Epidurally Administered Morphine

An epidural block with neurolysis is seldom used because it does not usually give satisfactory results. However, a sacral epidural block can be very effective in cases where pain in the perineum and other well-defined areas is not helped sufficiently by other methods.

As mentioned in Chapter 1, there are morphine receptors in the spinal cord, which are found mainly on the primary afferent nociceptive pain neuron and on the ascending neuron (see Fig. 10). Morphine therefore inhibits the transmission of pain impulses in the spinal cord.

In the 1970s, studies in which morphine was administered intraspinally or epidurally to animals yielded the following results among others:

1. Small doses (one-tenth of the size of intramuscular doses) provided very good pain relief.
2. The effect lasted much longer than that of intramuscular injection.
3. There was no motor or sensory impairment, and the animals' movements were quite normal.
4. No changes were registered in autonomic functions such as blood pressure, pulse, and respiration.
5. No observable changes were noted in the animals' behavior, in contrast to the behavior observed after systemic use of morphine.
6. The animals did not develop abstinence symptoms, even after long-term treatment.

These results were so promising that spinal and epidural administration of morphine was tried on humans, and in 1979 the first findings were published. The results in humans were analogous to those in animals. A dose of 2–6 mg morphine administered epidurally provided good pain relief, which lasted from 4 to 24 hours. There were few side effects, although a few patients did develop intensive itching or urinary retention. These favorable results led to immediate widespread use of the method, and soon reports began to come in of the serious side effects. Severe respiratory depression could occur as late as 12 to 24 hours after the last dose, and several deaths were reported, usually in patients with acute pain, such as after surgery. However, in cancer patients being treated for chronic pain by this method, respiratory depression has been extremely rare. The reason why the respiratory depression occurs after such a long time is that epidurally administered morphine is distributed throughout the cerebrospinal fluid, and it takes several hours to reach and depress the respiratory center. It should be noted that part of the injected morphine is absorbed by the epidural veins and thus has systemic effects. Further, because of the circulation of the cerebrospinal fluid, the morphine concentration in the brain may be considerable, although it is substantially less than that found with the systemic morphine therapy required to give the equivalent pain relief.

The method is very suitable for cases where systemically administered analgesics either have not been effective or have had unacceptable side effects.

A permanent epidural catheter is introduced and tunneled subcutaneously for 10–20 cm to avoid infection in the epidural space (see Fig. 33). The catheter can be used for several months, and in some cases for over a year. The morphine can be injected by the patient, the patient's family, or a visiting nurse. The ordinary dose is 4–10 mg morphine four to six times a day, but considerably higher doses often have to be used. The morphine is diluted in isotonic saline to a total volume of 5–15 ml. If the morphine does not provide effective relief on its own, a local anesthetic such as bupivacaine can be given as well. This is usually given for types of pain that do not respond well to morphine.

This method is a great step forward in the treatment of cancer pain and has enabled many patients who had previously been suffering intolerable pain to live a fairly normal life.

SYMPATHETIC BLOCK

Visceral pain is conducted mainly along nerves from the sympathetic nervous system and can therefore be relieved by sympathetic blocks. Pain transmitted by somatic nerves will also sometimes respond to a sympathetic block, since in certain cases the norepinephrine secreted from sympathetic nerve endings in the tissue causes pain in the injured nerve structures. Causalgia and other neuropathic pain can sometimes be relieved effectively by a block of the sympathetic nervous system.

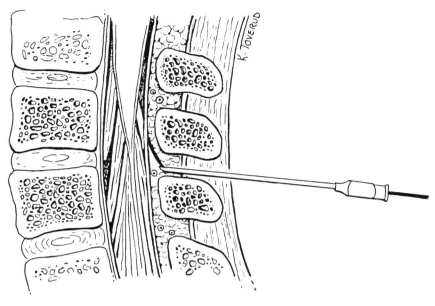

FIGURE 33. Positioning of an epidural catheter. The epidural needle is inserted between two spinous processes, e.g., L_2 and L_3. When the tip of the needle is in the epidural space, the catheter is inserted and the needle removed.

Block of the Celiac Plexus

The visceral nociceptive fibers mainly follow the pathways of the sympathetic nervous system, and blocking the sympathetic ganglions will therefore provide good pain relief. The pain fibers from the upper region of the abdomen pass through the celiac plexus, a network of fibers and ganglia surrounding the aorta and the vena cava at the level of the first lumbar vertebra. A block is indicated in cancer of the upper part of the abdomen (the stomach or the pancreas) that causes visceral pain and/or nausea that is not relieved by peripherally acting analgesics or compound analgesics in adequate doses. The block should be done before the patient requires large doses of opioids and while the patient's general condition is reasonably good.

The insertion is made just below the twelfth rib. A prognostic block with a local anesthetic is usually done first, and if this is successful a therapeutic block with ethanol, 50%, is carried out afterward or the next day.

The most common side effects are temporary orthostatic hypotenion and diarrhea, both due to the reduced sympathetic tone.

The block is very effective in most cases, and the pain relief lasts for a few weeks to half a year. The block can be repeated, and it also alleviates nausea from local causes.

Stellate Ganglion Block (see Fig. 34)

The stellate ganglion is the uppermost ganglion in the sympathetic trunk and supplies the head, neck, upper thorax, parts of the upper limbs, and parts of the visceral thoracic organs. The ganglion is situated just in front of the transverse process of the seventh cervical vertebra. The ganglion can be blocked by inserting a needle medial to the carotid artery at the level of the sixth or seventh cervical vertebra. Local anesthetic is used, and the block is repeated as necessary. Neurolytic agents are not usually suitable because they would give the patient a permanent Horner's syndrome.

Lumbar Sympathetic Block (see Fig. 35)

When a sympathetic block is indicated to alleviate pain in the pelvis and lower extremities, the sympathetic trunk can be blocked in the lumbar region. Usually a diagnostic block with a local anesthetic is done first, by

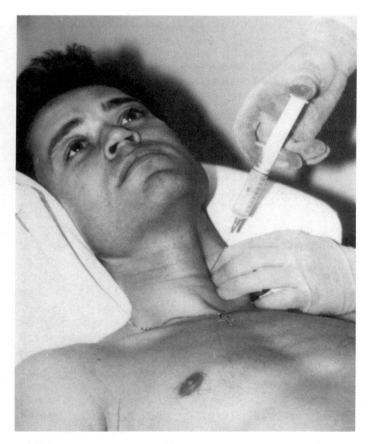

FIGURE 34. Stellate ganglion block.

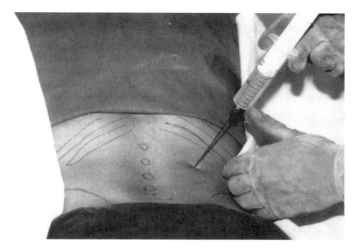

FIGURE 35. Lumbar sympathetic block.

inserting needles paravertebrally on one or both sides. The needles are moved forward until the tips reach the anterolateral side of the vertebral body. Here, too, the effect of repeated blocks with a local anesthetic can last for a long time, and more long-lasting relief can be obtained by injecting a neurolytic solution or by surgical sympathectomy.

Intravenous Sympathetic Block in the Extremities

Guanethidine releases the neurotransmitter norepinephrine from its storage sites in the peripheral sympathetic nerve fibers and also blocks the reuptake of norepinephrine. When these terminals have been emptied it takes a long time for them to resynthesize the transmitter substance. At the same time the guanethidine acts as an antagonist to norepinephrine at receptor level and inhibits the action of the remaining neurotransmitter. When guanethidine is injected into the tissues, its high affinity causes it to remain there for several days, up to 3 weeks according to some measurements. The effect of the first injection usually lasts 3 to 7 days, but after repeated injections the effect may last even longer. See Fig. 36.

Guanethidine is injected intravenously into an extremity that has been previously "emptied" of blood. A tourniquet cuff inflated to 50–100 mm Hg above the arterial blood pressure will prevent new blood from entering the extremity. After the guanethidine has been injected it should be allowed to work for about 15–30 minutes, during which time it will bind strongly to the tissue, so that only a small fraction will enter the systemic circulation after the cuff has been deflated.

The block may be very effective for neuropathic pain in, for example, causalgia or allodynia. In addition to alleviating the pain, the block causes

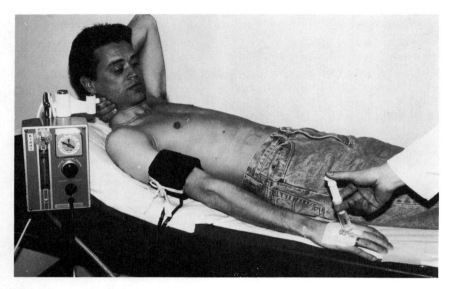

FIGURE 36. Sympathetic block with guanethidine administered intravenously in an extremity emptied of blood.

an increase in the peripheral circulation. It is therefore also suitable for vasospastic pain (Raynaud's disease) and other conditions involving reduced circulation. The injection should usually be repeated at 3 to 7 day intervals at first and later at longer intervals. The block is also worth trying for phantom pains and has been reported to have a reasonably good effect on pain caused by central nervous system injuries after cerebral stroke or intracranial tumors. The mechamism behind this is not clear.

NEUROSURGERY

Many neurosurgical techniques can provide effective relief from pain, but they are often very expensive in terms of resourses, so rather few patients are able to benefit from them.

Percutaneous cordotomy is one of the commonest methods. The ventral spinothalamic tract is severed at the level of the first and second cervical vertebrae, and this reduces the perception of pain and temperature on the contralateral side of the body. The other sensory and motor pathways are retained. The operation is usually done under local anesthesia. It is indicated in one-sided pain, is effective in the majority of cases, and is used when other methods have proved ineffective. Possible complications are hemiparesis and respiratory insuficiency. The pain usually returns after 6 to 12 months and may take the form of very painful neuralgia in the part of the body that was previously supplied by the severed nerve fibers. This is the main reason why it is performed only on patients with a short life expectancy.

Destruction of the Pituitary Gland has been shown to provide long-term relief, especially in cancer of the breast and prostate with skeletal metastasis. The technique consists of injecting 1 ml of ethanol into the pituitary gland. This is not enough to destroy its function completely, but the ethanol probably triggers the production of substances that alleviate pain (possibly endorphins). The method is indicated in cases of bilateral cancer pain that is not relieved by adequate drug therapy. The relief may last for several weeks to a year or more. During the procedure the ethanol may spread beyond the pituitary gland and affect the optic nerve, resulting in blindness. If it spreads upward to the hypothalamus and the third ventricle, it may cause death. Proper drug therapy, if necessary with an epidural catheter, makes it very seldom necessary to carry out such a destructive technique on the central nervous system.

Dorsal Column Stimulation resembles transcutaneous electrical nerve stimulation in its mode of action. Instead of stimulation through the skin, the stimulus is applied electrically directly into the epidural space. This increases the analgesic effect and enlarges the area affected. The method consists of implantation of permanent electrodes in the epidural space, which can be stimulated by a small electric, battery-operated device that can be attached to the patient's body.

Research is being done on the implantation of electrodes in various parts of the brain, and some of the results have been promising. These methods will probably be used a good deal in the future.

TRANSCUTANEOUS ELECTRICAL NERVE STIMULATION (TENS) AND ACUPUNCTURE

TENS and acupuncture are gaining ground in medical circles, mainly because they have been investigated scientifically and shown unequivocally to relieve pain in many cases. See Fig. 37.

It is thought that these methods stimulate the body's endogenous pain-inhibiting mechanisms (see Chapter 1). High-frequency TENS (50–100 Hz) probably utilizes spinal gate control. The effect is rapid and ceases relatively soon after the stimulation is withdrawn. Low-frequency TENS (2–5 Hz) and acupuncture are thought to liberate various substances including beta-endorphins. Naloxone often blocks the effect. The analgesic effect is evident after 20–30 minutes and may last for several hours after the treatment is over.

Acupuncture involves the insertion of needles into the skin at certain points; the needles may be moved about or electrically stimulated or may remain still. The technique requires very thorough training.

TENS is done by attaching two or four electrodes to the skin and

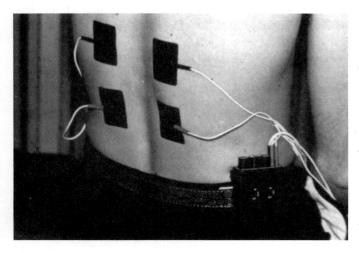

FIGURE 37. Transcutaneous electrical nerve stimulation.

stimulating them by means of a small battery-driven apparatus the size of a pocket calculator. The stimulation may be at a high or low frequency. At a high frequency (50–100 Hz) the patient feels a prickling or tickling sensation on the skin. The strength of the current is adjusted so that it can easily be felt without being painful. High-frequency stimulation must be done in the area of the pain or close to it, or on the opposite side of the body. If the stimulation takes effect, it usually does so fairly rapidly. With this type of stimulation the placing of the electrodes is very important, and they often have to be placed in different positions before a good effect is obtained. It is a good idea to let the patient find the best position for the electrodes. With low-frequency stimulation (2–5 Hz), the position of the electrodes is less important, because this type of stimulation probably does not activate the spinal gate control in the same way and may act by liberating endorphins and other humoral substances. To obtain relief from pain with low-frequency TENS the stimulation must be strong enough to cause muscular contraction but not so strong that the contractions cause pain. It usually takes about 15–30 minutes before the patient feels any pain relief, but the effect can last for several hours after the stimulation has ceased. With both these methods the usual procedure is stimulation for 30 minutes two to three times a day, but this varies considerably. With high-frequency TENS, for example, some patients require almost continuous stimulation, while others only need 15 minutes once a day.

There are no clearly defined indications for the use of acupuncture and TENS in the treatment of pain in cancer. Most studies of the direct application of these methods to cancer pain have not shown very positive results. But it is quite possible that certain subgroups of cancer patients may benefit from them, especially those with pain in the musculoskeletal system or the skin or with neuropathic pain. About 50–60% of all patients with chronic pain experience some relief with these methods, and with chronic treatment about 30–40% usually continue to feel relief. The methods usually prove ineffective if combined with opioid therapy, and they should be started at a relatively early stage of the disease. When carried out *lege artis*, their side effects are few and harmless. TENS is contraindicated in patients with on-demand pacemakers because these machines can interpret the electrical current as a heartbeat and thus as a signal to stop their action.

9

Methods
of Treatment
that Reduce the Size
of the Tumor

PALLIATIVE SURGERY

For a patient with a poor life expectancy, surgery is indicated only if it can increase the patient's well-being by lessening pain or alleviating other unpleasant or distressing symptoms.

GASTROINTESTINAL TUMORS
THAT CANNOT BE RADICALLY REMOVED

In cases of manifest intestinal obstruction an ileostomy or colostomy is often performed even if there is demonstrable metastasis. It is, however, possible to control the symptoms of gastrointestinal obstruction without surgery in the terminal stage (see p. 173). As much as possible of the primary tumor should be removed to reduce future growth into the abdominal wall, nerve plexuses, or other abdominal organs. This can save the patient from a great deal of pain and suffering. Removing as much as possible of the tumor also facilitates radiotherapy because it reduces the target volume. This in turn reduces the side effects because a smaller area is irradiated. In cases of obstruction in the sigmoid colon or rectum, laser surgery with a colonoscopic technique is a gentle and effective method of widening the passage.

Obstructive cancer of the esophagus can be very unpleasant because the patient is unable to eat or drink and in extreme cases to swallow saliva. Insertion of a tube into the esophagus can make a great deal of difference to the patient's well-being, and it is often done in spite of the potential complications. Laser surgery is now frequently used to clear the obstruction.

Jaundice caused by cancer obstructing the bile ducts sometimes gives rise to unbearable itching. In such cases surgical drainage of the ducts can help the patient immeasurably.

SKELETAL METASTASIS

In cases of radiologically verified skeletal metastasis and where there is a risk of fracture, radiotherapy should be given. If the risk of a fracture is very high, however, it is worth performing a prophylactic internal fixation, which can save patients a good deal of pain and can be done when they are in reasonably good health.

Active treatment is required for pathological fractures due to tumor infiltration. Internal fixation relieves pain effectively in 90% of patients and leads to growth of the fracture in many cases. Many patients need radiotherapy at the same time. Without surgical treatment every movement is painful, but internal fixation means that the patients are more mobile and more able to take care of themselves, so that they can avoid institutional care.

SKIN METASTASES

Skin metastases should be removed at an early stage so that they do not develop into large necrotic tumors, which are very unpleasant for patients, their families, and the nursing staff.

PALLIATIVE RADIOTHERAPY

The aim of palliative radiotherapy is to alleviate the symptoms by means of the smallest possible doses and the lowest possible number of fractions.

PAIN RELIEF

Radiation can be very effective in treating painful skeletal metastases. The pain can be relieved completely and the effect may last for several months, which may delay or avoid the use of strong analgesics. The effect depends on the radiation sensitivity of the tumor and the position of the metastasis, but relief from pain can be obtained even with fairly insensitive tumors.

Radiotherapy is most suitable for one or a few painful areas. Sometimes effective radiotherapy directed against the most painful areas reveals pain in other areas, but the latter usually responds well to ordinary analgesics.

In cases of widespread metastasis with many areas of pain, a single dose of 6–8 Gy directed at the upper or lower half of the body may give good results. If necessary, a similar dose can be applied to the other half of

the body 6 to 8 weeks later. This procedure can provide good and prolonged pain relief, but it is not without side effects and should be restricted to patients with severe pain that has responded poorly to conventional treatment.

Patients with painful tumors in the central nervous system, pancreas, liver, and lungs, soft-tissue metastases, and infiltrating tumors in
nerve tissue (e.g., epidural, in a large nerve plexus, or in peripheral
nerves) can also benefit from palliative radiotherapy.

Some patients experience increased pain after the first few treatments, due to reactive edema. The pain can be lessened by means of
glucocorticosteroids and patients should be warned of this possibility beforehand so that they do not lose faith in the treatment.

Side effects occur seldom with the small doses used for palliative
treatment, except for the half-body irradiation, which can result in a distressing amount of nausea and vomiting.

PALLIATIVE TREATMENT OF OTHER SYMPTOMS

Ulcerating skin tumors are very unpleasant and very distressing for the
patient and surroundings, and radiotherapy should be considered. This
can considerably reduce the size of a sensitive tumor, and the skin may re-
form.

Dyspnea and cough caused by bronchial carcinoma can be alleviated
by irradiation in doses that do not give severe side effects.

PALLIATIVE CYTOSTATIC THERAPY

If there is hope of a cure or remission, high doses of strong drugs are
worth trying in spite of the strength of the side effects, but for palliative
treatment lower doses or less toxic drugs are used. The difference between
therapeutic and toxic doses of cytostatic drugs is very small, however, so
this type of treatment always involves a continual balancing act between
improving the patient's condition and preventing the occurrence of serious side effects.

PAIN RELIEF

Pain is often caused by solid tumors and their metastases, and cytostatics
often have little effect on these types of tumors, especially during the later
stages of the disease, when resistance may develop to drugs that have
been used for some time. Hematological tumors frequently respond better,
with a considerable lessening of the pain, but here, too, the effect diminishes as the disease progresses. A number of studies have been carried out
on the palliative effects of cytostatic therapy, but most of them have not
evaluated the effect of pain. It is thus difficult to obtain a clear picture of
the role of cytostatics in pain relief on the basis of the available publica-

tions, and cytostatics are seldom used to treat pain unless it is thought that they will also affect the course of the disease.

ENDOCRINE THERAPY

Cancer of the breast and prostate, adenocarcinoma of the uterus, leukemia, lymphoma, and cancer of the thyroid can be influenced by endocrine therapy because they often possess estrogen and gestagen receptors (cancer of the breast, uterus), androgen and estrogen receptors (cancer of the prostate), or cortisol receptors (leukemia, lymphoma). Endocrine therapy cannot effect a cure, but it can relieve symptoms and has relatively few side effects. The response, however, may not be apparent until after 4 to 6 weeks of treatment.

PAIN RELIEF

Most studies investigating pain relief by means of endocrine therapy have dealt with small, heterogeneous groups of patients, and the pain-relieving effect has not always been carefully evaluated. However, clinical evidence clearly indicates that hormone treatment can be effective against pain.

Cancer of the prostate with painful metastases. The primary aim of any treatment here is to reduce the level of testosterone, because this can affect the growth of the tumor. The most common solution is orchiectomy (removal of the testes), because this often provides effective pain relief and has few side effects. The testosterone level can also be lowered by administration of estrogens, but this increases the frequency of cardiovascular disease in men. An alternative treatment is to administer a luteinizing hormone-releasing hormone (LH-RH) antagonist, either alone or together with an antiandrogen. The effect may not be apparent for the first 4 weeks or so, and the patient may even suffer more pain at first. If these methods have not had the desired effect the next step to combat the pain from metastasis is usually irradiation. In cases of widespread metastasis pain can be relieved by treatment with prednisone in doses of less than 30 mg per day, usually in the form of four doses a day in order to obtain a continuous suppression of the endogenous hormone production from the adrenal cortex. Medroxyprogesterone acetate can be given instead of, or in addition to, prednisone. If there is widespread skeletal pain in spite of adequate pain therapy, half-body irradiation can be considered.

Cancer of the breast with metastases. The treatment of choice for receptor-positive tumors is administration of tamoxifen, an effective antiestrogen with few side effects. The effect is potentiated if medroxyprogesterone acetate is given as well. Prednisone also usually has a satisfactory effect on pain caused by skeletal metastasis. Sometimes hormone therapy is tried on receptor-negative tumors for palliation and alleviation of pain, because some of these patients do respond to it. But generally receptor-negative tumors are subjected to cytostatic treatment, such as with doxorubicin, 20 mg per week. Sometimes the production of sex hormones in the adrenal cortex in breast cancer can be stopped by administering aminoglutethimide. Occasionally there may be indications for half-body irradiation or injection of ethanol into the pituitary gland if the pain is intractable.

Medroxyprogesterone acetate has a certain pain-relieving effect in cancer of the breast and prostate and hypernephroma. The dose is 300 to 1500 mg per day (usually 600–1000 mg), and the result can be seen within 1 to 4 weeks. The drug also has a certain anabolic effect. In higher doses it can give rise to weight increases, edema, Cushing's syndrome, and vaginal bleeding. Some patients also suffer from nausea and dyspepsia.

All investigations of endocrine therapy have reported that the number of patients experiencing pain relief is considerably higher than the number of objective remissions, measured in terms of tumor reduction. A number of patients have less pain in spite of the fact that their disease is progressing. The pain relief afforded by endocrine therapy is therefore to some extent independent of the antineoplastic effect.

The place of endocrine drugs in the treatment of pain has been much discussed. Generally speaking, these drugs ought to be restricted to patients with other indications for hormone treatment, or to cases where other methods of pain relief have been tried without success.

OTHER FORMS OF PALLIATION

Most hormonal preparations have a certain anabolic and tonic effect that benefits the patient.

PART III

PRACTICAL APPLICATIONS

10

Practical Application of Pain Treatment

The different types of pain respond very differently to analgesics, so that before beginning the treatment it is essential to assess the pain correctly. Generally speaking, deep-seated, aching, nociceptive pain from soft tissue, musculoskeletal system, and visceral organs responds well to analgesics. Ordinary analgesics have a limited effect, however, on pain triggered by movement, certain types of neuropathic pain, and colic. If the pain diagnosis is correct, the response to treatment can often be predicted and an effective alternative can be used if strong analgesics are not expected to have a good effect (see also Table 7 on p. 85 and Chapter 2, p. 27–30).

Treatment should be started as soon as the pain becomes a problem for the patient. There is no reason to fear that the drugs will become less effective with time, since the dosage of a morphinelike drug can be increased according to need without necessarily increasing the side effects. In the terminal stage it is therefore easier to help patients who have received proper analgesic therapy during the course of their disease than those who have not been adequately treated. The patient should become used to receiving help for pain and not have to bear it for as long as possible. Regular prophylactic pain therapy should therefore be started at once, according to a schedule and not as required (p.r.n.). This means that the next dose of analgesic is given before the previous one has ceased to take effect, so that the patient is assured of relief from pain day and night. As far as possible the drugs should be given by mouth and in large enough doses. Finally, one of the most important factors in the successful treatment of pain is to have regular contact with the patient and continually reevaluate the response to the treatment. Cancer is a chronic process and the pain will often vary considerably during the course of the disease, making it necessary to readjust dosages and alter treatment strategies.

MILD TO MODERATE NOCICEPTIVE PAIN
ADMINISTRATION OF ANALGESICS

Treatment is started with peripherally acting analgesics in sufficiently large doses:

Aspirin, 0.5–1.0 g × 4–5 (6)
Acetaminophen, 0.5–1.0 g × 4–5 (6)

The figures in parentheses represent the number of doses that may be suitable for certain patients.

These two drugs are obtainable as tablets and in liquid form. Debilitated patients may find the mixture easier to take. The size of the dose should be adapted according to the patient's requirements, and there is no need to restrict the dosage unless large doses produce undesirable side effects.

If the above medication is not sufficient, a combination can be tried, in the form of aspirin or acetaminophen and one of the following:

Codeine, 30–60 (100) mg × 4–5
Propoxyphene chloride, 70–140 mg × 2–4
Propoxyphene napsylate, 100–200 mg × 2–4

Some NSAIDs (aspirinlike drugs) are as effective as the above combinations against pain from musculoskeletal tumors, and it can be an advantage to try them before starting on codeine or propoxyphene because they have no sedative effect. Further, they do not produce side effects such as dizziness and confusion, nausea is less of a problem, and constipation is rare. The disadvantage of these drugs is that they affect the hemostatic system and are contraindicated for patients with peptic ulcer, although they have less influence on the gastric mucosa and on clotting than aspirin has. The NSAIDs generally used in such cases are:

Diflunisal, (250–)500 mg × 2
Naproxen, 250–500 mg × 2
Ibuprofen, 200–600 mg × 3–4
Sulindac, 200 mg × 2

These drugs can also be effectively combined with codeine or propoxyphene to increase the analgesic effect.

If a combination of drugs is chosen, the dose of each component should be checked to see that it is large enough (see p. 100). Many of the commercially available compounds do not fulfill this requirement.

Pharmacologically, codeine combines well with aspirin, acetaminophen, or ibuprofen, all of which have similar half-lives and duration of action. Propoxyphene combines well, pharmacologically speaking, with diflunisal or naproxen. Propoxyphene is available in tablet form, usually combined with acetaminophen or aspirin, although the propoxyphene component has a longer half-life than either of the two latter components. Initially the components have a similar duration of action because the long duration of action of propoxyphene is built up by repeated doses, as with methadone. Chronic use of propoxyphene involves a risk of accumulation, especially of its metabolites, although in practice this is rarely seen with doses of less than 600 mg per day. Thus the combination of propoxyphene and acetaminophen or aspirin usually functions well.

It is often preferable to use a free combination of a peripheral and a centrally acting analgesic rather than a fixed combination in one tablet. This is mainly because tolerance develops to the centrally acting component (codeine/propoxyphene/morphine, etc.), and the dose has to be increased with time in order to maintain the effect. Peripherally acting analgesic will remain, while that of the centrally acting analgesic will gradually decline. Thus a patient taking, for example, acetaminophen combined with codeine on a long-term basis will continue to benefit from the acetaminophen but not from the codeine, although the latter will retain its constipating effect. With free combinations, however, the doses can be increased independently to achieve a maximal effect.

The recommended doses of codeine and propoxyphene have an analgesic effect that corresponds to that of 0.5–1.0 g of aspirin, and they cannot be regarded as strong analgesics. This also applies to pentazocine in tablets of 50 mg.

OTHER MODES OF TREATMENT

Alternatives to the use of systemic analgesics should be considered at an early stage. If they are successful they may delay or avoid the use of opioids.

Radiotherapy can have a very good effect on pain from skeletal or soft-tissue metastases or tumors that press on nerve structures, and good pain relief can be obtained even with relatively radioresistant tumors. The dose of radiation can usually be divided into a few fractions, and since the irradiated area is usually small this normally limits the side effects. In certain cases half-body irradiation can have a good effect on the pain from widespread skeletal metastasis. Radiotherapy should therefore be considered for all painful localized tumors (see p. 126), especially skeletal metastases (see p. 147).

Nerve blocks. Peripheral nerve blocks can be used when the pain is restricted to a limited area and where the blocking of the nerve will not destroy important motor functions. With pain in the upper abdomen, for example, caused by cancer of the stomach or pancreas or metastasis to the liver, blocking of the celiac plexus can provide long-lasting relief from pain and nausea. Pain in the pelvis or lower limbs can be an indication for a subarachnoid phenol block, but in recent years such patients have generally been given epidural morphine treatment. Both these methods are described in detail in Chapter 8.

Neurosurgery is usually of limited value, but percutaneous cordotomy is worth considering for patients in a great deal of pain who have not responded to analgesic or any other therapy. This operation presupposes that the patient's pain is restricted to one half of the body and that the life expectancy is less than a year (see p. 120).

Transcutaneous electrical nerve stimulation (TENS) and acupuncture can be tried with patients suffering from musculoskeletal or neuropathic pain at a relatively early stage of the disease.

Hormones and cystostatics may be used in certain selected patients to relieve pain (see pp. 127–129).

Even after opioid therapy has been started, other methods should always be taken into consideration.

SEVERE PAIN

For oral medication in severe pain, morphine and methadone are usually the drugs of choice, and when properly used these two drugs are nearly always effective. Alternatives are hydromorphone, levorphanol, and buprenorphine. It is perfectly possible to relieve very severe pain by oral medication, without recourse to injections, provided that the medication is given regularly and before the effect of the previous dose has worn off and that large enough doses are used. The dosage should therefore be regulated according to the effect on the patient. Considerably higher doses than for acute pain are often necessary, and the metabolism of the drug (especially the first-pass metabolism) shows marked individual differences, so that the same dose of morphine can give differences in plasma concentration by a factor of up to 5 in different patients (see Table 8 on p. 89).

Most patients prefer oral therapy in the form of tablets, but a drug in liquid form has some advantages:

1. It can be taken even if there is difficulty swallowing.
2. The opioid content can be altered without altering the volume of the mixture.
3. The vehicle can be altered according to taste.

The volume of liquid should be 10–20 ml per dose, which means that the opioid content can be varied from 5 to 100 mg as necessary. The opioid can be mixed with almost anything, but if the mixture is to last for over a week it should contain a preservative, such as spiritus conservans, 1–4%.

CURRENT PAIN MIXTURES

A current pain mixture is:

Purified water, 100 ml
Morphine or methadone, 1–2–5 mg/ml

This mixture can be given with or without flavoring, such as black currant syrup, which disguises the rather bitter taste of morphine. Chloroform water may be used instead of ordinary water, to take away some of the bitter taste. Ordinary injectable solution can be used, mixed with black currant juice and water. Commercial oral solutions of morphine and methadone are also available in the United States.

If a neuroleptic is to be given as well, it can be added to the solution as drops or the opioid can be added directly to an already available liquid neuroleptic.

When a patient is nauseated by the medication, it is important to find out whether the nausea is caused by the taste of the solution or by the pharmacological effects of the drug. If nausea and vomiting occur immediately after taking the medication, they are usually due to additives in the mixture. Nausea due to absorbed morphine or methadone is not generally felt until about a half-hour after the medicine has been taken. Different-tasting vehicles should be tried, but once nausea has been felt, patients often continue to be nauseated by a mixture even if the taste is changed. Many of them stop feeling sick after changing to tablets, so that this should be done if possible.

MORPHINE OR METHADONE?

In most cases both these drugs are equally effective, although very severe pain seems to be relieved better by morphine. The side effects, which vary considerably between individuals, usually determine which drug should be used. (See Table 12.)

Because of its long duration of action, requiring less frequent doses, and the danger of accumulation, *methadone* is most suitable for:

Ambulant patients.
Patients with fairly constant (not fluctuating) pain.
Patients in reasonably good health.

Morphine is preferable for:

Fluctuating pain, because a steady state is rapidly achieved and it is easy to increase the dose.
Treatment of debilitated patients, because they can easily be overdosed with methadone and become very sedated.
Very severe pain.

TABLE 12. Morphine or Methadone?

Morphine	Methadone
Advantages	Advantages
Easily controlled	Long-lasting effect, pain relief all night
Rapid achievement of steady state	Infrequent dosage, easy to use for
	ambulant patients
Little danger of accumulation	
Flexible, dosage can be adapted to daily	
pain variations	
High doses possible for severe pain	
Can be given to elderly and debilitated	
patients	
Disadvantages	Disadvantages
Frequent dosage[a]	Danger of accumulation, with sedation
	and confusion
Pain at night	Less flexible
	Less suitable for very severe pain

[a]This problem has now been solved by the introduction of slow-release tablets with an 8–12-hour duration of action.

HOW TO FIND THE CORRECT DOSE

There are great individual variations in the bioavailability of the various opioids. The same oral dose can give plasma levels up to five times higher in one patient than in another. Standard doses of opioids are just as unsuitable for all cancer patients as standard doses of insulin are for all diabetics (see Table 9 on p. 90).

The art of good pain treatment is to use doses that are high enough to give the patient good pain relief but not so high as to constitute overdosage, resulting in, for example, strong sedation.

Morphine

Two to three times as much morphine is generally required to obtain the same effect orally as parenterally. The usual initial dose is 5–20 mg of morphine by mouth, depending on weight, age, pain intensity, and previous use of a centrally acting analgesic. Thus, elderly patients usually start with 5 mg; younger patients who have previously taken fairly large doses of codeine or propoxyphene would require 10–20 mg from the beginning. Right from the first the drug should be given every 4 hours, or more often if necessary. If the pain has not been adequately relieved after two to four doses, the dose should be increased by 50%, and if a good result is not obtained after two to four more doses, the dose should again be increased by 30–50%, and the procedure repeated until the pain is adequately relieved. The patient should be carefully followed up the first 2 or 3 days, so that the right dose can be found as quickly as possible. The treatment should then be reassessed twice during the following week. A dosage of 5–50 mg every 4 hours is enough for most patients, but doses of 100 mg or more are not uncommon. High doses can be used as long as the patient's pain requires, since pain is the best antidote to the side effects of morphine.

Slow-release morphine tablets are now available, with a duration of action of 8–12 hours, so that they need to be taken only two to three times a day. This is easier and more pleasant, and it allows the patient to have a whole night's sleep without pain. Morphine treatment is generally started with ordinary tablets or a mixture every 4 hours for several days to establish the necessary dosage, after which the required 24-hour dose can be given in the form of slow-release tablets.

Methadone

Frequent doses are necessary for the first 1 to 3 days because methadone has a long duration of action and does not take effect until the concentration in the body has reached a steady state. This can be done in several ways.

It has been recommended to give 5–10 mg every 4 to 6 hours the first day followed by 10 mg once a day, on the basis of a mathematical assessment of the pharmacokinetics. If this does not provide relief, 15–20 mg every 6 hours for a day followed by the same dose once a day can be tried.

I usually recommend a patient-controlled regimen. The patient is given an initial dose of 5–10 mg methadone and instructed to take a new dose as soon as the pain returns and increases in intensity. This is repeated as often as required, so that continuous relief is obtained from the first day. At first the patient often takes large daily doses, but usually the interval between doses is gradually increased. After a week the physician prescribes an 8-hour interval between doses, and the size of the dose is regulated by the amount used by the patient during the previous day. This method ensures rapid and effective relief from pain, while keeping the risk of overdosage and accumulation to a minimum. It also gives the patient an active role to play in the treatment, which in itself is valuable.

Most workers involved in treating pain in cancer patients consider it clinically advisable to give methadone in small doses two to four times a day rather than in one large dose. If a single large dose is chosen, it is best given in the evening, when the sedative effect can be utilized while the plasma level is at its peak. The usual daily dose is 20–40 mg, varying from 10 mg to over 100 mg.

Buprenorphine Sublingual Tablets

These are useful when the patient has difficulty in swallowing. Studies indicate that the analgesic effect is similar to that of morphine or methadone for many patients. Buprenorphine seems to have more side effects, but this is highly individual. The usual dosage is one to two sublingual tablets (0.2–0.4 mg) every 4 to 6 hours, and this can be increased to 1.2 mg at the same intervals. Long-term use of sublingual tablets can give rise to sores in the mouth.

Hydromorphone

This is given orally according to exactly the same principles as morphine. Hydromorphone, 2 mg, usually corresponds to morphine, 10 mg.

PROBLEMS IN CONNECTION WITH OPIOID THERAPY

Side effects are relatively common, especially at first, but usually they are not so severe that the treatment has to be discontinued, and they can often be alleviated by other drugs.

Respiratory Depression

When strong analgesics are given in accordance with the patient's need for pain relief, respiratory depression is not a problem in practice, even if the doses are very much higher than normal. This is because the pain stimulates the respiratory center and thus counteracts the inhibiting effect of the opioid. Tolerance to the respiratory depression develops faster than the tolerance to the analgesic effect. Depressed respiration is thus not a problem in the treatment of chronic pain in cancer, but care should be taken if opioids are given in combination with other medication that depresses the central nervous system, especially during the initial phase of the treatment.

A number of patients with pain associated with cancer also have chronic lung diseases like bronchial asthma or emphysema. The respiratory center of such patients often has a reduced sensitivity to carbon dioxide, and they are more susceptible to respiratory depression in connection with morphine than other patients. In practice, they can usually be treated for pain in the same way as patients with healthy lungs, and respiratory depression is extremely rare in connection with oral therapy in these patients. They must be carefully followed up and psychotropic drugs should be avoided in combination with the opioid medication.

If respiratory depression does occur, it should be treated by intravenous injection of naloxone, starting with a very small dose: one ampule of 0.4 mg diluted to 10 ml with saline solution. The best method is to inject 0.1 mg (2.5 ml) at a time and wait 1/2 to 1 minute to see the effect. The dose can be gradually increased until the patient no longer has depressed respiration but still has pain relief. If a large dose is given at once, the patient may experience severe abstinence symptoms, which are very unpleasant. The duration of action of naloxone is not much more than an hour, and the dose may need to be repeated. If the patient is overdosed with methadone the effect will last a long time because of the long half-life of methadone, and naloxone may have to be administered several times.

Methadone is more rapidly excreted from the body in acid urine, so that the effects of overdosage can be shortened by acidifying the urine with ammonium chloride or large doses of, for example, vitamin C.

Sedation

With the correct dosage the patient is sedated for the first 2 to 5 days. This is due partly to the sedative effect of the drug and partly to the fact that the relief from pain causes the patient to relax, perhaps for the first time for a long period. After this initial phase the patient becomes more alert and can remain completely so even with large doses of opioid. Patients and their families should be warned about the initial sedative effect; otherwise they often think that the disease has become worse, and some patients stop taking the medication because they are afraid of becoming permanently sedated.

If the patient is still drowsy after 5 days of treatment with the same dose, this may be due to the following:

1. Overdosage.
2. Simultaneous use of psychotropic drugs, especially low-potency neuroleptics (chlorpromazine and methotrimeprazine), antidepressants, and benzodiazepines.
3. Advanced disease with accompanying lethargy and sedation.

The sedation can be treated by discontinuing or reducing the dose of the other drugs or, if appropriate, of the opioid. In rare cases the use of a psychostimulating drug is indicated—for example, cocaine, 5–20 mg two to four times a day, with the highest doses taken early in the day.

Confusion, Disorientation, and Hallucinations

Up to 10% of patients develop these symptoms, most frequently the elderly and debilitated. Confusion and disorientation are usually dose dependent, while hallucinations can also occur at lower doses. The side effects can be treated by reducing the dose, changing to a different centrally acting drug, or supplementing with a neuroleptic (see Chapter 11, p. 161).

Dizziness and Unsteadiness

These symptoms occur most frequently in elderly patients and may be due to postural hypotension or a disturbance of the vestibular system. They are dose dependent.

Tolerance

The development of tolerance means that when a drug is used over a long period the dose has to be increased in order to achieve the same effect. This is a normal biochemical process that occurs with all centrally acting analgesics. Such drugs are widely believed to lose their analgesic effect after a time, but this does not in fact happen. With the right dosage adequate pain relief can be given through all the phases of a disease. Tolerance develops most rapidly during the first weeks of therapy, but after this point the same dose can often be used for a long time. With some patients the dose can even be reduced as they approach the terminal stage. Tolerance also develops much more quickly with intramuscular and especially with intravenous therapy than with oral therapy. If the pain is of the type that only partly responds to opioids or if the experience of the pain is largely influenced by emotional, social, or existential factors, the dose often needs to be increased fairly rapidly. But naturally it is always possible that an increase in dose is required because of an aggravation of the disease with increased pain.

Nausea and Vomiting

These reactions are less frequent in bedridden patients, but are relatively common in ambulant ones. They can complicate oral therapy, especially because they may make the patient reject it and ask for injections. Some patients are nauseated by the taste of the mixture; in such cases the nausea is felt immediately after or while the patient is taking the dose. If the nausea is an effect of the opioid it arises about half an hour after the dose has been taken. It is often wise to administer an antiemetic prophylactically, especially to ambulant patients. However, the nausea often diminishes after a while and may become less pronounced as the dose is increased. Some patients, on the other hand, do not feel nauseated until some time after they have begun taking the drug. Pain can also give rise to nausea, which is sometimes eliminated by strong analgesics. Nausea may also be caused by the cancer itself.

See also a more detailed treatment of nausea in Chapter 11, p. 167.

Constipation

Patients on long-term therapy suffer from severe constipation, and all patients receiving treatment with centrally acting analgesics should take laxatives regularly (see p. 171).

Effect on the Urogenital Tract

Predisposed people may develop urinary retention from morphine or similar drugs. This is rare, however, except in connection with epidural morphine administration. A few patients develop urgency incontinence.

Sweating

Some patients suffer from distressing sweating, especially at night.

Dryness of the Mouth and Nose

This develops in a certain number of patients, especially if they are taking drugs with anticholinergic effects, such as meperidine.

The treatment for all the above side effects is dealt with in Chapter 11.

TREATMENT OF PAIN IN PATIENTS WHO CANNOT TAKE ORAL MEDICATION

SUPPOSITORIES OR RECTAL SOLUTION

Morphine and meperidine are available as suppositories, and the rule of thumb is to use the same dose for rectal as for oral administration. Suppositories are often a good alternative when a patient cannot take medication orally for some reason, but the disadvantage is that absorption from the rectum varies a great deal, depending on whether there are feces present. Rectal solutions, which a pharmacy will make up to the necessary strength, are an alternative. It is a good idea to add methylcellulose to rectal solutions, so that they do not run out so easily.

PARENTERAL INJECTIONS

Intramuscular or intravenous injection should be a last resort for cancer patients, to be avoided as far as possible. This method means that the patient has to be injected every 4 hours around the clock over a long period. Pharmacologically speaking, too, injections are an undesirable form of treatment for chronic pain, since they cause the plasma level to rise rapidly, often to a point where the patient is slightly overdosed and consequently sedated. After this the level sinks, also fairly rapidly, so that the duration of action of an injected drug is usually shorter than that of an orally administered one (see p. 52). Other methods should therefore always be tried first.

CONTINUOUS SUBCUTANEOUS INFUSION

The recent introduction of this method of administration has been a great step forward in the treatment of cancer pain. The drug is administered by means of a drug delivery pump (Fig. 38), a small battery-driven device either with a mechanism that regularly depresses the plunger of a syringe containing an analgesic, or with a medication reservoir (cassette). The dose can be regulated by altering the speed. A thin catheter leads from the pump to a butterfly needle attached subcutaneously to the abdomen or thorax. In this way a slow continuous infusion of morphine is administered (see Fig. 39). The syringe usually needs to be filled once a day, while the medication cassettes last longer and need to be filled every 2 to 7 days. The advantage of this method is that it gives the patient uninterrupted analgesia with only very small changes in the plasma concentration. Consequently, the side effects like sedation and nausea are often less pronounced, and the patient avoids repeated injections. A butterfly needle

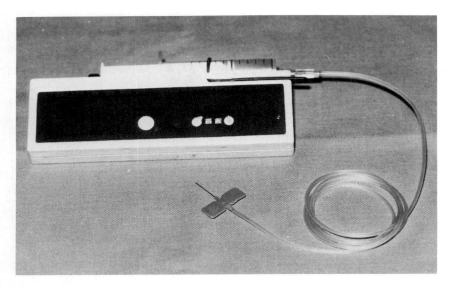

FIGURE 38. Drug delivery pump.

can be used for up to 3 weeks, but if there are signs of infection or infiltration it has to be changed more often. Only morphine, hydromorphone, heroin, and buprenorphine can be used in a drug delivery pump because the other strong analgesics usually irritate the tissue too much. The patient's movements are not impeded in any way by a pump, which fits into a small shoulder bag or a carrying pouch that can be worn beneath the clothing.

The use of a drug delivery pump is indicated for patients who cannot take oral medication because of nausea, vomiting, or difficulties in swallowing and for patients who need high doses of analgesics that cannot easily be administered in any other way. It is often useful in the terminal stage, when other methods of administration can be very difficult.

If the pain suddenly increases in intensity, an incremental dose can be given. A drug delivery pump is so simple that an ambulant patient can usually be taught how to use it. A visiting nurse can also help.

CONTINUOUS INTRAVENOUS INFUSION

Continuous intravenous infusion may be an alternative for bedridden patients in the terminal phase who cannot take oral medication. The required amount of analgesic is mixed with a suitable amount of infusion solution for 24 hours, and the drip is regulated according to the need for analgesia.

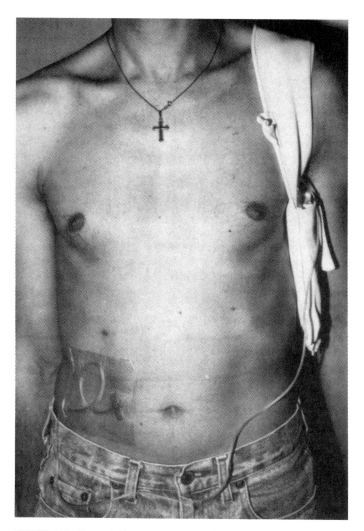

FIGURE 39. Drug delivery pump worn by a patient in a shoulder bag, with the butterfly needle attached subcutaneously on the abdomen.

EPIDURAL MORPHINE ADMINISTRATION

Epidural administration of morphine can be a very good method of treating patients with severe pain who cannot take oral medication or who do not obtain sufficient relief from it. A catheter is inserted in the epidural space, tunneled subcutaneously for 10–30 cm, and connected to a bacterial filter (see Figs. 40–41). This method requires much lower doses of morphine than are necessary for oral or subcutaneous administration, so the patient usually experiences less sedation or nausea. The analgesic effect is

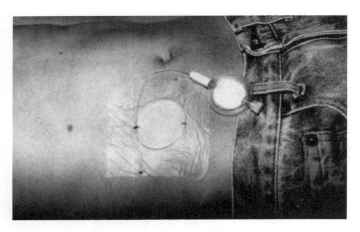

FIGURE 40. Closeup of an epidural catheter attached to a bacterial filter. The catheter is tunneled subcutaneously around the flank.

strong. The usual dose is 4–20 mg of morphine every 4 to 6 hours, but some patients require much higher doses. Better relief, especially from the sharp, neuropathic type of pain, is obtained if the local anesthetic bupivacaine, 0.125–0.5%, is given in addition to morphine. The usual volume for epidural administration is 5–15 ml. When bupivacaine or some other local

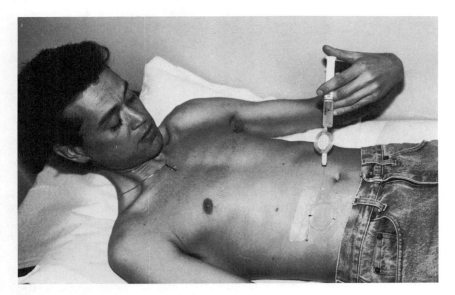

FIGURE 41. A patient learning to inject morphine into an epidural catheter.

anesthetic is given as well, the catheter should be inserted at the level of the spinal segment corresponding to the area of the pain.

The patient or a family member can be taught to inject the morphine two to six times a day, or the patient may prefer to have a visiting nurse do it. In some cases the drug delivery pump is coupled to an epidural catheter that provides a continuous infusion of the drug. This is usually employed for the administration of local anesthetics, since these drugs have a rather short duration of action when injected. If the catheter is correctly positioned and no infection arises, it can remain in place for several months. A number of patients have had treatment lasting 1 or 2 years by this method. A more detailed description is given in Chapter 8.

TREATMENT OF PAIN CAUSED BY A NEOPLASM

SKELETAL METASTASES

The first step is to consider whether the lesion(s) is suitable for radiotherapy or whether there are indications for cytostatic or hormone therapy. Metastasis to long bones may require internal fixation by surgery in order to prevent fracture.

Clinical studies have shown that inhibitors of prostaglandin synthesis (NSAIDs, aspirinlike drugs) have a beneficial effect and provide good pain relief in most patients, since prostaglandins can contribute to osteolysis and pain in skeletal metastases. One can therefore begin treatment of pain from skeletal metastasis by administering NSAIDs, usually diflunisal (250–)500 mg × 2; naproxen 250–500 mg × 2; sulindac, 200 mg × 2; or ibuprofen, 200–600 mg × 3–4.

Glucocorticosteroids also have a good effect on pain from skeletal metastases, because they reduce the edema surrounding the tumor and also because they effectively inhibit prostaglandin and leukotriene synthesis and thus have a directly analgesic effect. They inhibit pain indirectly in castrated patients with tumors sensitive to sex hormones because of the negative feedback effect on ACTH and the subsequent reduced production of sex hormones by the adrenal cortex. Prednisone/prednisolone or dexamethasone is most commonly used. The usual dosage of prednisolone is 10–30 mg per day, in one to four doses; four doses are necessary if the production of sex hormones needs to be suppressed for the whole 24 hours. Dexamethasone is useful if a strong anti-inflammatory effect combined with a minimal mineral corticoid (fluid-retaining) effect is required. Dexamethasone, 1 mg, corresponds to prednisolone, 5–7 mg. The treatment is started by giving 4 mg two to four times a day and keeping the patient on this dosage until pain relief is obtained. The dosage is then reduced over 1 to 2 weeks to the level of 1–4 mg once a day. This high-dose treatment often provides very good pain relief. The combination of an NSAID and a glucocorticosteroid has an additive effect in relieving pain and can be used when indicated, but the incidence of side effects on the upper gastrointestinal tract is significantly increased. It may be a good idea to give an antacid, a receptor histamine H_2 blocker, or sucralfate as a prophylactic measure.

Some studies have shown that calcitonin given in doses of 100 IE (1 ml) intramuscularly once a day can have a good effect on pain from skeletal metastasis, usually in the course of the first week.

Hypercalcemia is a not uncommon complication of skeletal metastasis (see Chapter 11, p. 180) and is very painful for the patient. This can be combated by all the drugs mentioned above, since they lower the calcium levels, but here again the response is individual. If the calcium levels are not reduced with NSAID, steroids or even calcitonin should be tried.

A new treatment option for hypercalcemia and painful skeletal metastases is provided by the diphosphonates clodronate and ethidronate, each of which directly or indirectly inhibits osteoclast function. They can be given orally and have few side effects, but we have little experience of these drugs as pain relievers.

If none of these drugs provide adequate relief, additional opioid therapy should be given, as described above (p. 138).

COMPRESSION / INFILTRATION OF NERVES

As mentioned in Chapter 2, compression and/or infiltration of nerves can give rise to several different kinds of pain. Compression can cause deep-seated, aching pain and also superficial, radiating pain. Infiltration often provokes superficial burning pain and allodynia. Sometimes sharp, shooting, radiating pain occurs in the area supplied by the nerve. Deep-seated, aching pain associated with compression can be helped by opioids, but usually not superficial burning pain, which requires other methods. Pain from compression and infiltration of nerves can be difficult to treat, and several methods often have to be tried.

Medication

Glucocorticosteroids often have a good effect on pain from nerve compression or infiltration, possibly because they reduce the edema surrounding the nerve structures. The usual treatment is 10–30 mg of prednisolone per day. Sometimes a stronger remedy is necessary, generally 4 mg of dexamethasone four times a day, gradually reduced to 2–4 mg per day over 1 to 2 weeks.

Opioids are often necessary, especially for deep-seated, aching pain. These should be administered as described above (p. 138).

Sharp, paroxysmal radiating pain can be helped by *antiepileptic drugs*—for example, carbamazepine, 200 mg two to four times a day, or sodium valproate, 150–300 mg three times a day. Starting with a low dose and increasing gradually will help reduce the side effects. It may take up to a week to reach the full effect.

Some patients with neuropathic pain, especially superficial burning pain, respond well to *tricyclic antidepressants,* in doses well below the level used to treat depression. There are exceptions, however, who need high doses for pain. The pain is usually relieved within 3 to 7 days after the therapeutic dose has been established. Amitriptyline is the usual choice, with an initial dosage of 10–25 mg two hours before sleep. The dose is increased by 10–25 mg every second night until the patient is sleeping better and experiencing pain relief. At therapeutic doses the patient usually has a more or less dry mouth but should not be distressingly sedated during the day. If the patient responds, relief from pain is usually obtained at doses of <75 mg a day. Some patients do better on three doses a day than on one. Other alternatives are imipramine and doxepin. Sometimes an increase in dosage to 75–150 mg per day over 1 to 2 weeks can be tried, but it is a good idea to escalate the doses fairly slowly to reduce side effects.

Radiotherapy

Radiotherapy often has a good effect, but radiation injury or fibrosis around the nerve can aggravate the pain in the long run.

Nerve Blocks

If one or only a few peripheral nerves are compressed or infiltrated, repeated blocks with local anesthetic, if necessary combined with a glucocorticosteroid into or near the lesion, can be tried. The effect sometimes lasts longer than the pharmacological properties would lead one to expect. If the local anesthetic block has a good but brief effect, a permanent neurolytic block of the affected peripheral nerves can be considered. The advantages of such a block should always be weighed against the possibility of paresis, and it should be given only to patients with a limited life expectancy.

If the compression or infiltration is more widespread—for example, involving nerve plexuses—an epidural block may be indicated. The most usual method in recent years has been epidural administration of morphine, but movement-related, stabbing, lancinating pain and superficial burning pain generally do not respond well to morphine alone, and here a local anesthetic like bupivacaine, 0.125–0.5%, can be given epidurally in addition. The effect on pain lasts only 1 1/2 to 3 hours after the injection, so continuous infusion by means of a drug delivery pump is often the best solution.

If the effect of epidurally administered morphine and/or bupivacaine is not satisfactory, a subarachnoid phenol block should be considered. It can be very effective and when done properly the risk of an unintentional paresis is relatively small.

Neurosurgery

Percutaneous cordotomy may have a good effect on pain at rest and with movement, but this method should be used only with patients with a short time to live, generally speaking not more than a year. Neurectomy and rhizotomy should also be considered.

GROWTH INTO HOLLOW ORGANS OR DUCTS LEADING FROM VISCERAL ORGANS

The indications for surgery must be evaluated in each case on the basis of the patient's general condition and life expectancy. Even patients with advanced disease will often tolerate a palliative operation, which can give them considerable relief. This applies, for example, to intestinal obstruction, which can be relieved by stoma; obstruction of the bile ducts, which can cause intense and distressing itching; and obstruction of the urogenital tract, which can cause pain and sometimes uremia. Neurolytic block of the celiac plexus can alleviate pain for several months.

In terminal patients, gastrointestinal obstruction can be controlled without surgery and often without resorting to a nasogastric tube. The parenteral administration (preferably by continuous subcutaneous or intravenous infusion with a drug delivery pump) of sufficiently large doses of an opioid such as morphine, combined with an antiemetic (e.g., haloperidol) and a spasmolytic (scopolamine), can give the patient much relief. See also Chapter 11, p. 173.

STRETCHING OF MEMBRANES AND CAPSULES SURROUNDING ABDOMINAL ORGANS

Cancer of the liver, pancreas, and other abdominal organs causes stretching of the membranes and capsules around the organs. Neurolytic blocking of the celiac plexus can give complete relief from pain over a long period in such cases (see p. 117).

Glucocorticosteroids (e.g., prednisolone, 10–30 mg per day) can alleviate pain through their antiedematous action. Aspirin sometimes helps pain from cancer of the pancreas. Intra-arterial infusion of cytostatics to the affected organs has been reported to have a good effect on pain, but the indications for this are very rare.

Opioids generally have to be prescribed for this type of pain, and they are usually effective if given by mouth or epidurally.

COMPRESSION / INFILTRATION OF BLOOD VESSELS

Arterial occlusion leading to ischemia may necessitate the surgical insertion of a graft, but this is very rarely done.

Edema of the extremities caused by disease of the veins or lymph vessels is best treated by elastic bandaging and elevation of the affected part and, if necessary, physiotherapy or treatment with an antiedema pulsator. Diuretics are also worth trying, although they are seldom effective. Injections in the affected limb should be avoided because of the danger of infection.

If a tumor causes pressure on blood vessels, as in edema in the head and neck caused by obstruction of the superior vena cava or edema in the legs caused by growth into the pelvis, surgery or radiotherapy should be considered.

High doses of glucocorticosteroids (e.g., dexamethasone, 4 mg four times a day) may cause the tumor to shrink, allowing a freer passage of blood. Compression or infiltration of blood vessels is often accompanied by venous thrombosis, which requires anticoagulation therapy, and this in turn complicates the treatment of pain because NSAIDs and glucocorticosteroids increase the risk of hemorrhage.

If none of these methods provides effective relief, opioids should help. Epidurally administered morphine may be a good alternative in cases of edema in the extremities.

SOFT-TISSUE INFILTRATION

The pain from infiltration in soft tissues can often be helped by surgery or radiotherapy. When neither of these is possible a nerve block or epidurally administered morphine can be effective if the position of the tumor is suitable.

The first drug to try is an NSAID such as diflunisal or naproxen. If this does not give satisfactory relief, an opioid can be added, as described above (pp. 136–140). Glucocorticosteroids such as prednisolone, 10–30 mg per day, may reduce the pain and should be tried if the above methods have failed. Infiltration in skin and mucous membranes can give rise to ulcerating tumors that may be painful. Here again peripherally acting analgesics, if necessary combined with opioids, are generally successful. Such tumors are often infected by bacteria and fungi and need proper local treatment or even systemic antibiotics. This is described in more detail in Chapter 11. Tricyclic antidepressants, especially amitriptyline, can help superficial burning pain.

HEADACHE CAUSED BY INCREASED INTRACRANIAL PRESSURE

With an intracranial tumor there is, of course, always a case for evaluating the utility of surgery or radiotherapy. Intrathecal or intra-arterial infusion of cytostatics is occasionally helpful.

If none of these forms of treatment are practicable, and the intracranial pressure needs to be reduced, steroid treatment with dexamethasone should be given, starting with 4 mg four times a day for 3 to 7 days and then gradually reducing the dose to the smallest possible maintenance dose. The patient's condition determines any further alterations in dosage.

TREATMENT OF PAIN CAUSED BY CANCER THERAPY

PAIN FOLLOWING SURGERY

Nerve Injuries

A nerve injury can cause permanent changes in the form of small nerve sprouts or neuromas. These are hypersensitive to touch and to norepinephrine. The pain is aching and burning, sometimes with paroxysmal, lancinating pains triggered by small movements. Ordinary analgesics are seldom effective with this type of pain, and drugs that have been shown to have a good effect are antiepileptic drugs such as carbamazepine, 200 mg two to four times a day, or sodium valproate, 150–300 mg two to three times a day. A good many patients with superficial burning pain and allodynia respond to antidepressants like amitriptyline or imipramine, 25–75 mg per day.

Transcutaneous electrical nerve stimulation should be tried at a relatively early stage of the disease. First high-frequency stimulation is applied to the painful area or just beside it. This helps some patients; others have more pain, and they can try stimulation of the opposite side of the body. If this does not help, low-frequency stimulation can be tried, with a strong enough current to cause muscle contraction. This is carried out in an area adjoining the painful area or on the hand.

Nerve blocks sometimes alleviate this type of pain. These consist of repeated blocks with a local anesthetic, combined with glucocorticosteroids injected directly into the painful area containing the neuromas and scar tissue. An epidural catheter may be tried, but these patients usually have a relatively long life expectancy, which limits the use of this method. For the same reason, neurolytic blocks are very seldom used, because they can cause paresis and sometimes permanent neuropathic pain. In some cases cryoanalgesia is effective.

Three pain syndromes are relatively common after surgery—postthoracotomy pain, postmastectomy pain, and pain after radical neck dissection (see p. 41). Usually the injury involves several nerves, but after mastectomy some patients have an injury to the intercostobrachial nerve only. Repeated blocks with a local anesthetic and, if necessary, steroids can relieve the pain for short or long periods.

In some patients the pain from nerve injuries can be improved by a sympathetic block and this should always be tried for unrelieved pain, although only a fraction of patients are helped. In some cases a new operation is indicated, but this often provides short-term relief or none at all.

Pain after Amputation

Pain in the stump is often due to scar shrinkage and the formation of neuromas. Palpation of the painful area will often reveal excessively tender spots, and repeated injections of a local anesthetic together with depot steroids in these spots is usually very effective. If the pain is very distressing a corrective operation should be considered, although such operations fail to relieve the pain amazingly often. It is important to make sure that the prosthesis fits properly and does not press against the painful areas, or does so as little as possible.

Phantom pains are also sometimes due to neuromas. The stump should be palpated for points that trigger the phantom pain when pressed. If there are such points, the pain can be helped by repeated injections of a local anesthetic and a steroid. In many cases, however, there are no such points, and other treatments have to be tried. Transcutaneous electrical nerve stimulation sometimes helps, and in some cases blocking of the sympathetic trunk helps. Reoperation often has very little effect. Irreversible forms of treatment like phenol blocks and destructive neurosurgery should be avoided. Some patients are helped by dorsal column stimulation (see p. 121).

Drug therapy for this type of neuropathic pain is the same as that described above. Some patients, but probably only a few, respond well to a combination of amitriptyline and morphine or methadone. If there are indications for the use of centrally acting analgesics in these patients, in spite of the fact that they have a normal life expectancy, the treatment should be carried out as described on p. 155.

Adhesions

Abdominal surgery sometimes results in the formation of adhesions, which give unpleasant symptoms like colic and indigestion. Corrective surgery should be considered but will often cause new adhesions and is thus not always very effective. Laxatives, especially products that soften the stools, should be given, and anticholinergic therapy can be tried. Small doses of loperamide, one to three tablets a day, also seem to help. The indications for analgesics, especially the centrally acting type, are very limited, except in patients with a short life expectancy.

Patients with chronic pain following surgery can be very difficult to treat. Many of them have been cured of their cancer by the surgery but they may have to live with the pain for years. The main guidelines for treatment are to try all the local treatments described above and, if necessary, administer peripherally acting analgesics and antidepressants. Centrally acting analgesics like codeine, propoxyphene, and morphine should be avoided in these patients because they are not very effective and in these cases they may easily be misused because of their psychological effects (sedation, relief of anxiety).

PAIN FOLLOWING CHEMOTHERAPY

Painful Polyradiculoneuropathy

Painful polyradiculoneuropathy is often due to treatment with *Vinca* alkaloids and/or cisplatin. The symptoms usually disappear when the treatment is discontinued, but not always. In the latter cases the pain is usually in the extremities, and these patients may be helped by intravenous administration of guanethidine (sympathetic block; see p. 119) and a tricyclic antidepressant taken by mouth.

Steroid pseudorheumatism is treated with small doses of steroids that are gradually reduced.

Herpes Zoster and Postherpetic Neuralgia

The treatment of pain in acute herpes zoster depends on the patient's age and immune status. For immunocompetent people under the age of 50, prednisone, 60–80 mg per day for 7–10 days, is recommended, together with a centrally acting analgesic. Recent studies indicate that treatment with systemic acyclovir (an antiviral drug rather specific for herpesviruses) is effective against pain and shortens the acute attack. Somatic and sympathetic nerve blocks can have a good effect if carried out at an early stage and may reduce the duration of the attack. Some studies suggest that they reduce the risk of developing postherpetic neuralgia. The block may be in the affected nerves or in the epidural space. Some patients respond well to TENS. These methods should be supplemented by amitriptyline in increasing doses up to a maximum of 75–100 mg per day over 1 to 2 weeks. Carbamazepine may help against paroxysmal, lancinating pain and should be given in doses of 200 mg two to four times a day. Sometimes up to 1200–1600 mg a day may be necessary, as long as side effects do not prevent this.

Patients with immune suppression caused by drugs or by disease should be given systemic acyclovir (Zovirax), an antiviral drug specific against herpesvirus. Early nerve blocks and treatment with analgesics, amitriptyline, and/or carbamazepine should be employed as described above.

Postherpetic neuralgia can be very difficult to treat, and most methods are not very effective. Studies have shown that amitriptyline can relieve pain in doses of 50–150 mg per day. Treatment is started by giving doses of 25 mg in the evening and gradually increasing the dose until the desired effect is obtained. At this dose the patient also develops dryness of the mouth, should sleep well, but should not be unpleasantly sedated during the day. Sometimes the therapeutic effect can be increased by combining the amitriptyline with fluphenazine, 1–2 mg three times a day. Carbamazepine should be used for paroxysmal, lancinating pain as indicated above. Sympathetic blocks and repeated subcutaneous injections with a local anesthetic and a steroid in the painful areas can also help.

Transcutaneous electrical nerve stimulation should also be tried. The effect is usually poor if the painful area is directly stimulated because it contains sensory deficits, but neighboring areas or the opposite side of the body can be used. If high-frequency stimulation has no effect, low-frequency stimulation of a neighboring area or of the hand can be tried.

A number of patients respond well to centrally acting analgesics, and if the pain is severe the use of opioids over a long period can be justified even if the patient has a relatively long life expectancy. Drugs with the longest possible duration of action should be given (methadone, MS Contin) and in the lowest possible doses. The prescriptions should always be issued by the same physician and the same pharmacy should be used every time. This situation presupposes a relationship of trust between the physician and the patient, who must not be allowed to increase the dose without first consulting the physician. In these cases centrally acting analgesics should be combined with amitriptyline to keep the dose of the former as low as possible.

Many patients with postherpetic neuralgia have secondary pain in the muscles and bones and benefit from physiotherapy and trigger point injections.

Postherpetic neuralgia is a chronic and painful disease, which requires holistic treatment. As much as possible should be done to avoid a chronic pain syndrome, including preventive measures against psychological and social complications. Such patients therefore often need multidisciplinary therapy.

PAIN FOLLOWING RADIOTHERAPY

During and immediately after the acute phase of radiotherapy local edema may arise and cause pain. This can be alleviated or prevented by glucocorticosteroids such as prednisolone, 30 mg or more per day. Pain that arises long after the end of the treatment can be caused by tissue fibrosis and scar shrinkage with constriction of nerves. This will develop into neuropathic pain, which can be treated in the same way as other neuropathic pain (see above).

Radiation treatment of the abdomen can cause chronic diarrhea and sometimes colic, which should be treated primarily by regulating the passage of stools. Anticholinergic drugs can help against the pain, and loperamide has been shown to alleviate the colic and reduce diarrhea.

PAIN CAUSED BY INACTIVITY AND CONFINEMENT TO BED

Bed-ridden patients often have pains in the musculoskeletal system. A long period in bed involves stretching of the muscles and ligaments as well as muscular atrophy and osteoporosis caused by inactivity. These pains should be treated primarily by physical measures such as regular changes of position in bed, active and passive movement of muscles and joints, and massage. Injections of local anesthetic, if necessary combined with glucocorticosteroids, in particularly painful areas such as ligament attachments and muscular trigger points are often helpful and sometimes remove the pain completely if done correctly. Inactivity and confinement to bed cause some patients to feel pain all over the body, but this responds to ordinary peripherally and centrally acting analgesics.

TREATMENT OF PAIN IN CHILDREN WITH CANCER

Cancer is fortunately rare in children but is still the second most frequent cause of death in childhood in the Western world.

Childhood cancer often starts with pain, but as soon as the child starts treatment, whether it takes the form of surgery, radiotherapy, or chemotherapy, the pain usually disappears. Ordinary analgesics generally help against the pain. The principles of treatment are the same as for adults (see below).

Anxiety and fear are closely connected with the experience of pain in adults and even more so in children. It is therefore extremely important to make the child feel as secure as possible during the initial stages of examination and treatment, in order to minimize the pain experience. The child has to go through a number of uncomfortable and frightening procedures such as blood sampling, insertion of an intravenous catheter, and bone marrow biopsies, and the distress can be reduced if the child is told what is going to happen, if the parents can be present whenever possible, and if the procedure is carried out calmly and unhurriedly. Small children are fairly easily distracted, but not older ones. If care is not taken to make the procedure as easy as possible, the child will come to associate everyone in a white coat with pain, and this will contribute to lowering the child's threshold toward fresh pain. Children who experience a lot of pain during the initial examination and treatment seem to have a lot more pain during the terminal phase as well. Thus preventive measures against pain early in the disease can reduce pain later. Narcosis should be used liberally for diagnostic procedures and operations; it has few side effects as a rule and is very useful in preventing anxiety and pain.

The pain caused by *advanced disease* is treated in principle in the same way in children as in adults. It is important to identify the type of pain and how far it is influenced by anxiety and insecurity. This can be difficult in small children, but continual crying, unhappiness, withdrawal, a tendency to isolation, and a lack of interest in playing often indicate pain. Even older children may have difficulty in distinguishing between feelings of pain, fear, insecurity, and so forth. But a child who says he or she is in pain should be taken seriously and given proper treatment. The same principle applies here as with adults: it is better to prevent the occurrence of pain than to treat pain that is already present. This means that medication should be given at regular intervals, usually not p.r.n. The intervals should be so short that the new dose is given before the old one has worn off, and the doses should be large enough to give proper relief. The size of the dose shows the same individual variation in children as in adults.

A peripherally acting analgesic can be used for mild to moderate pain, preferably acetaminophen, since the metabolism of this drug differs very little between younger and older children. The half-life is 2 1/2 to 3 hours, and there are usually few side effects. The normal dose is 60–80 mg per kilogram per day divided into four doses. Acetaminophen is available in liquid, tablet, and suppository forms. Aspirin is a good alternative and gives as much relief as acetaminophen. It is not advisable, however, for children undergoing cytostatic therapy because of the increased bleeding tendency. Ordinarily aspirin has little effect on the gastrointestinal tract in children. The dosage is 60 mg per kilogram per day in four doses. If the peripherally acting analgesic is not adequate, a combination of aspirin or acetaminophen and codeine or propoxyphene can be used.

If these compounds do not provide satisfactory relief, they should be replaced by stronger centrally acting analgesics. Methadone and morphine have been shown to give good results. The drug should be taken orally or in the rectum; only in exceptional cases should it be injected. Intravenous infusion can be used in the terminal phase, but only if there are other indications for infusion. An alternative is continuous subcutaneous infusion from a drug delivery pump, which usually works well and is not too uncomfortable for the child. A great many children, however, manage to take oral medication up to the last day before death.

As everyone knows, it can be difficult to get children to take medicine, so drugs that do not need to be taken often are to be preferred. Thus methadone is usually the drug of choice for severe cancer pain in children. It is normally given in liquid form but can also be given as a rectal solution or as a suppository. It is a good idea to add methylcellulose to the rectal solution to thicken it and prevent it from running out of the rectum so easily. As with adults, the dosage varies with the individual, and the doses should be given more frequently during the first 2 days than later. The usual dosage is 2.5–5 mg per m^2 body surface four times a day for the first 2 days and after that two to three times a day, but many children need higher doses. Methadone can also be combined with a peripherally acting analgesic like acetaminophen, in which case it can be given in the acetaminophen mixture. Methadone therapy can usually be carried out at home. The parents should be told to watch out for increased drowsiness and signs of withdrawnness, which can indicate overdosage. Some hospitals give the parents a dose of the methadone antagonist naloxone, to be administered intramuscularly or intravenously if an overdose should occur. This happens extremely rarely, however. If the child is treated at home the parents should be able to contact the hospital frequently so that they are sure of what they are doing and carry out the treatment correctly.

Morphine is an alternative to methadone but is more difficult to administer to children because the liquid form has to be taken every 4 hours. The slow-release tablets (MS Contin), which can be taken morning and evening, have altered this situation, however. A normal dose would be 5–30 mg per m^2 body surface per day, but here too the individual differences are large. The tablets must be swallowed whole if the effect is not to be lost.

The side effects should not be forgotten when treating children for pain. Constipation must be counteracted from the first day of administration of a centrally acting analgesic, by laxatives in the form of softening and peristalsis-stimulating agents, and enemas should be given whenever necessary. Metoclopramide is usually given for nausea in doses of 5–10 mg per m^2 body surface. Higher doses can be given, but there may be extrapyramidal side effects in the form of dystonia, which is more frequent in children than in adults. Antihistamines or neuroleptics may also help against nausea, but they are more sedating than metoclopramide. Some children experience itching when they take opioids, and local application of zinc liniment may help. If not, antihistamines can be given.

As I mentioned above, anxiety usually plays an important part in children's experience of pain. Tranquilizers (benzodiazepines) can be given liberally if they are necessary, but they should not be used as substitutes for the security and close contact that the child needs during the treatment.

11

Diagnosis and Treatment of Other Symptoms

Pain is not the only symptom that distresses cancer patients. Advanced cancer is a multiorgan disease with many different symptoms. These should be taken seriously and correctly diagnosed and treated.

SYMPTOMS FROM THE CENTRAL NERVOUS SYSTEM

ANXIETY AND MENTAL STRESS

Anxiety and distress are inseparable from the difficult situation of cancer patients. It is extremely important that the physician and nursing staff spend *time* with the patients and do what they can to relieve the anxiety. Patients must be given all the information they are entitled to and that they are able to absorb. Fear of the unknown is often much worse than definite knowledge of the facts of the disease. The same information will need to be repeated several times, and the patients must be allowed to express their anxiety and fear in connection with the progress of the disease, the future, their relations with their families, and so on. The family doctor is in a good position to help here, since he or she knows the patient's way of reacting, the family and home environment, and so on. Cooperation between the family doctor and the family, visiting nurses, social worker, priest, and others involved with the patient can make a great deal of difference and give the patient the all-round help that is needed.

Anxiety can be so distressing that it requires medicinal help. Benzodiazepines, taken regularly or as required, have a good effect, and addiction is not a problem in these cases. Oxazepam is eliminated effectively even when liver function is reduced, and since it has a relatively short half-life, it does not accumulate during chronic use. It is more slowly absorbed than the other benzodiazepines.

Neuroleptics and antidepressants also relieve anxiety, but many patients develop dysphoria after low-potency neuroleptics, so these should be used sparingly. Tricyclic antidepressants in doses of less than 75 mg per day often help to relieve anxiety and stabilize mood.

DEPRESSION

As with anxiety, comfort and support are essential when dealing with the natural sorrow and depression that accompany cancer. Symptoms of depression may be so pronounced that they need to be treated with antidepressants, especially since these drugs may also help relieve pain.

For patients with good general health who are not taking other medication affecting the central nervous system, the normal dose of a tricyclic antidepressant is 125–225 mg per day in one to three doses. After a cautious start of 10–25 mg one to three times a day, the dose is gradually increased over 1 to 2 weeks until the therapeutic dose appears to have been reached. The response to these drugs is very individual; some people can take up to 200 mg without any noticeable side effects like dryness of the mouth or sedation, whereas others become very sedated on doses of 25 mg per day.

If the general condition is poor and/or the patient is taking drugs that affect the central nervous system, the dose of antidepressant usually has to be reduced. These drugs can cause confusion in debilitated patients.

Low-potency phenothiazine neuroleptics can trigger or aggravate a depression and should be used with caution in connection with potentially depressive patients. Long-term opioid therapy can also cause depression.

If neuroleptics are indicated for such patients, the high-potency type should be used. Flupentixol, 0.5–1.5 mg in the morning and afternoon, and haloperidol, 0.5–2.0 mg two to three times a day, are probably the most suitable, since they often have a mildly stimulating and antidepressive effect. They combine well with an antidepressant like amitriptyline or doxepin, 25–75 mg in the evening. Dryness of the mouth can be a very uncomfortable side effect of tricyclic antidepressants. It is less pronounced for antidepressants like mianserin or trazodone.

In cases of *apathy* that do not respond to antidepressants or to a reduction in the dose of opioid, cocaine, 5–20 mg orally three to four times a day with the highest doses early in the day, can be tried. The dose must be adjusted so that the apathy is treated without mental confusion or hallucinations. Cocaine is very rarely used.

INSOMNIA

The first step in cases of insomnia is to try to find the cause, which may be something quite simple like the temperature of the room, noise, position in bed, and so on. Patients may also be kept awake by the medication they are taking, such as diuretics, sympathicomimetics, caffeine, glucocortico- steroids.

If the insomnia is caused by *anxiety*, the primary treatment is with a benzodiazepine preparation. Some studies suggest that meprobamate, promethazine, and barbiturates may excite patients with pain and aggra- vate the pain. This is probably an uncommon side effect, but it is worth bearing in mind when a hypnotic is prescribed. Many antidepressants have a sedative effect as well as relieving anxiety and are therefore very suitable for treating insomnia (see Table 10, p. 107). These drugs should be taken 1 to 2 hours before bedtime so that the patient can take advantage of the hypnotic effect without becoming too sedated the following day.

Pain at night should be treated by increasing the dose of analgesic until the pain is under control. Methotrimeprazine, 5–25 mg, can be given in addition since it has a strong sedative effect and may potentiate the analgesic. At first, low doses should be given before bedtime, because patients who are sensitive to methotrimeprazine can have nightmares and bad dreams.

Night sweating can disturb sleep considerably. It may respond to in- domethacin, 25–50 mg in tablet form or 100 mg as a suppository.

If a patient has recently begun treatment with strong analgesics, a strong hypnotic can easily have too sedative an effect, but after some time the risk of sedation decreases considerably.

CONFUSION

The diagnosis of confusion is sometimes based on inadequate grounds. Patients admitted to hospital are often entering a new and unknown envi- ronment. They are subjected to unpleasant and possibly frightening exam- inations and treatment. They are surrounded by new and difficult situa- tions and words and can easily become disoriented, especially if their sight or hearing is poor. This "disorientation" is not the same, however, as the psychiatric state of confusion.

Genuine confusion may be due to:

Cerebral injury (tumor, infarction).
Liver or kidney failure.
Hypercalcemia, hyponatremia.
Sepsis.
Drugs: opioids, psychotropic drugs, anticholinergics.
Senile dementia.
Severe depression.

Confusion is a serious diagnosis, and a thorough search must be made for the cause. This involves a neurological and general somatic examination and, if necessary, radiography, computed tomography, or a brain scan. Laboratory tests for liver or kidney insufficiency, calcium concentration, and drug levels in serum may be indicated.

The treatment should naturally be causal as far as possible. The patient should be helped to carry out practical tasks and the daily routine should be regular and organized so that the patient can take part in it and follow what is going on as far as possible.

If a drug is suspected to be the cause of the confusion, it should be reduced or discontinued. If cerebral hypoxia is indicated, oxygen treatment can be started. High doses of steroids are effective against confusion caused by a cerebral tumor. A patient who is disturbed and restless may be helped by diazepam or, even better, a neuroleptic in the form of haloperidol, 0.5–5 mg one to three times a day (little sedative effect), or methotrimeprazine, 5–25 mg one to three times a day (sedative effect).

GASTROINTESTINAL SYMPTOMS

DRY MOUTH

Dryness in the mouth and throat may be due to:

Drugs: anticholinergics, tricyclic antidepressants, neuroleptics, especially
low-potency phenothiazine derivatives, antihistamines, opioids.
Local radiotherapy.
Breathing through the mouth.
Dehydration.

The drug responsible for the symptoms is discontinued if possible. In the case of neuroleptics a high-potency preparation can be substituted, and if an antidepressant is needed, mianserin or trazodone can be used because they have little anticholinergic effect.

Symptomatic treatment primarily involves frequent and thorough care of the mouth. Sour-tasting drinks stimulate saliva production and moisten the mouth. The addition of methylcellulose gives a good mucous coating. Artificial saliva is easy to obtain and use and gives some relief. Cream mixed into the patient's drinks gives a pleasant mucous coating, and a mixture that is sometimes used consists of an egg, a tablespoon of sugar, and a tablespoon of cream lightly beaten together and mixed with fresh orange juice and ice cubes.

SORE MOUTH

A dry mouth may feel sore, but usually soreness of the mouth is caused by an inflammatory reaction due to:

Candidiasis (thrush) in the mouth.
Ulcerative stomatitis.
Malignant hematological disease.
Cytostatic therapy.
Local radiotherapy.

The candidiasis often appears as red inflamed mucous membranes, without the characteristic white plaques. It can be treated with nystatin oral solution, 1–2 ml every 4 hours, or clotrimazole oral suspension, 1–2 ml, or lozenges every 4 hours. If the candidiasis is severe and widespread and does not respond satisfactorily to local treatment, ketoconazole tablets for systemic treatment should be used. Two hundred milligrams one or two times a day for 10 days is usually adequate.

Ulcerative stomatitis and ulcers caused by cancer or its treatment can be treated with local lidocaine medication or steroid mouthwash/ointment.

NAUSEA AND VOMITING

We do not know the exact details of the physiological mechanisms behind nausea and vomiting. The medulla oblongata contains two relevant well-defined areas: the *chemoreceptor trigger zone (CTZ)* in the area postrema at the bottom of the fourth ventricle and the *vomiting center* anterior to this in the medulla near the vagus nuclei and the respiratory center (Fig. 42). The chemoreceptor trigger zone is not protected by the blood-brain barrier and

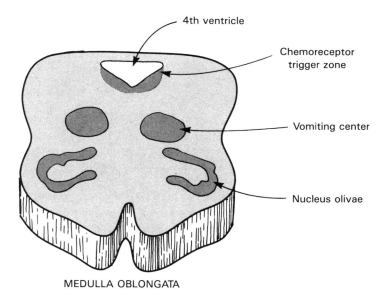

4th ventricle

Chemoreceptor
trigger zone

Vomiting center

Nucleus olivae

MEDULLA OBLONGATA

FIGURE 42. Vomiting center and chemoreceptor trigger zone in the medulla oblongata.

is thus easily affected by substances in the blood. Chemical substances in the blood are thought to be capable of causing nausea by affecting this zone. One of the neurotransmitters in the zone is dopamine, which acts on postsynaptic dopamine D_2 receptors. The vomiting center receives nerve impulses from sympathetic and parasympathetic nerves from the gastrointestinal tract, the vestibular nuclei, higher centers of the central nervous system and cerebral cortex, and the chemoreceptor trigger zone (Fig. 43). This center thus receives all the "emetic impulses" and, when sufficiently stimulated, gives rise to vomiting. Relevant neurotransmitters are acetylcholine and histamine, which act on muscarine cholinergic receptors and histamine H_1 receptors, respectively.

Causes

The causes of nausea and vomiting can be classified as follows.
Local conditions in the gastrointestinal tract:

Gastric irritation—for example, due to aspirin and other NSAIDs, glucocorticosteroids, cytostatics, alcohol, and antibiotics.
Reduced gastric emptying due to opioids, local tumor, liver or pancreas enlarged by a tumor.
Gastrointestinal obstruction.
Irritation of the pharynx.
Constipation.

Affection of centers in the brain stem, mainly the chemoreceptor trigger zone:

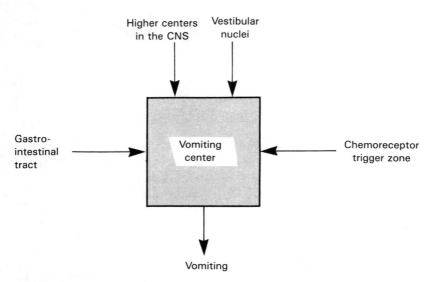

FIGURE 43. Afferent and efferent connections of the vomiting center.

Drugs: opioids, digitalis, cytostatics, estrogen.
Biochemical disturbances: hypercalcemia, uremia, liver failure.
Increased intracranial pressure.
Vestibular disturbance.
Systemic effect of cancer.
Radiotherapy.
Psychological/emotional factors.

Examination

It is important to find the reason for the nausea and vomiting so that the treatment can be as specific and rational as possible. The patient's history should include drug intake (opioids, NSAIDs, digitalis, cytostatics, hormones), previous episodes of nausea and vomiting, factors that improve or aggravate the nausea, possible constipation, and psychological factors. The clinical examination should include ophthalmoscopy to exclude the possibility of papillary edema, palpation of the abdomen, and rectal examination. The laboratory tests should include liver and kidney tests and electrolyte determination, especially measurement of the calcium content. See p. 180. If the patient takes digitalis, the level in serum should be measured.

Specific Treatment

Gastrointestinal causes. If there is a local tumor in the gastrointestinal tract or the liver and/or pancreas, surgery, radiotherapy, and cytostatic therapy should all be considered. Nausea due to tumor growth in the upper abdomen can be effectively relieved by a block of the celiac plexus (p. 177). Drugs that can cause gastric irritation (NSAIDs) or reduce intestinal motility (antidepressants, antipsychotics, opioids) should, if possible, be discontinued. It is important that any constipation be dealt with, since this is frequently a cause of nausea in cancer patients, especially if they are taking opioids.

Hypercalcemia is described on p. 180.

Increased intracranial pressure is described on p. 152.

Uremia. If the uremia is caused by an obstructed ureter, surgical correction is often indicated, in the form of an abdominal operation, insertion of a urethral catheter, or percutaneous nephrostomy. The last-mentioned operation can be carried out even on very ill patients, but in the terminal phase one is often faced with the choice of whether to prolong the patient's life by the operation or to "let nature take its course."

Symptomatic Treatment

Dopamine D$_2$ receptor antagonists. Dopamine is one of the neurotransmitters in the chemoreceptor trigger zone, and dopamine D$_2$ antagonists such as neuroleptics and metoclopramide alleviate nausea caused by chemical agents affecting this zone. This applies to nausea associated with medication, hypercalcemia, uremia, and so forth. Metoclopramide has little effect on nausea provoked by stimulation of the vestibular system, as in travel sickness and sometimes the use of opioids.

Metoclopramide counteracts nausea partly by its central action in blocking dopamine. It also increases the motility and speed of emptying of the stomach and small intestine, reducing the peripheral effects of nausea. Its effect on the motor action of the gastrointestinal tract is counteracted by anticholinergics. The side effects are drowsiness if used in high doses and, very rarely, acute dystonia. The latter can be treated with centrally acting anticholinergics. Domperidone has a similar mechanism of action to metoclopramide but does not cross the blood-brain barrier. Because of this, acute dystonia is very rarely seen.

Metoclopramide is available as tablets, suppositories, mixture, and in injectable form. It is easily absorbed in liquid and tablet form, less so as a suppository. The first-pass metabolism is very variable, and dose-dependent kinetics can occur at doses above 10 mg. The normal half-life is 2 hours, but with higher doses it may be longer. The duration of action is 1 1/2 to 3 hours. The recommended dose is 10 mg three times a day, but this can be increased if necessary to 10–40 mg four to six times a day if side effects do not prevent this. Sometimes considerably higher doses are used.

The antiemetic dose of a neuroleptic is low, so there are usually few side effects. During the day high-potency neuroleptics should be used because of their less pronounced unspecific sedative action; examples are haloperidol, 0.5–2.0 mg two to three times a day, and prochlorperazine, 5–10 mg two to three times a day. At night a sedative low-potency neuroleptic can be beneficial, such as chlorpromazine, 5–25 mg.

If the neuroleptic alone is not effective, it can be combined with metoclopramide. The local action of metoclopramide in the gastrointestinal tract will be counteracted by the strong anticholinergic effect of a low-potency neuroleptic, and an increased antiemetic effect is best achieved by combining metoclopramide with a high-potency neuroleptic (piperazine, phenothiazine, or butyrophenone). The risk of extrapyramidal side effects also increases, but these are so rare that in practice they do not constitute a contraindication. If they occur, they usually disappear rapidly when treated with a centrally acting anticholinergic such as biperiden, 5 mg intravenously, or orfenadine, 10 mg intravenously.

Anticholinergics. Acetylcholine is one of the neurotransmitters in the vomiting center, and anticholinergics can therefore reduce vomiting. Scopolamine has been shown to be effective against both nausea and vomiting, but its sedative and anticholinergic action usually limits its use. However, it can now be administered as a plaster on the skin, which reduces the side effects. Low-potency neuroleptics have an anticholinergic action that may potentiate the antidopaminergic, antiemetic effect.

Antihistamines that block the histaminergic H_1 receptor are particularly effective against nausea caused by movement and to some extent against nausea from other causes. The emetic effect of opioids may be related to disturbances in the vestibular system, since ambulant patients feel it most. This type of nausea can be helped by antihistamines. Most antihistamines also have some anticholinergic effects and can be combined with neuroleptics and/or metoclopramide. Hydroxyzine is often suitable for cancer patients with nausea, since it relieves the nausea in doses that are not large enough to have a sedative effect. It may potentiate the analgesic effect of opioids and is effective against pruritus. The usual dose is 10–25 mg one to four times a day.

Glucocorticosteroids. The nausea and vomiting associated with cytostatic treatment may be due to prostaglandins, and large doses of steroids have been reported to have a good effect. It has not been established whether this is due to inhibition of prostaglandin synthesis.

A number of cancer patients suffer from nausea even when neither hypercalcemia nor any other apparent cause can be found. Many of them do not respond well to ordinary antiemetics, but steroids sometimes help in these cases. The usual dose is 10–30 mg of prednisolone per day or corresponding doses of some other steroid (see Table 4, p. 77). Higher doses can sometimes be tried.

Opioids. Nausea due to pain is reduced by opioids, but opioids can also cause nausea. Nausea due to opioids may be reversed by naloxone, although in some patients naloxone has the opposite effect.

Antianxiety drugs can help against nausea by inhibiting conditioned reflexes, as in the nausea induced by cytostatic treatment.

Tetrahydrocannabinol (the active component of cannabis and marijuana) has been tested to see whether it can reduce nausea provoked by cytostatic therapy. Some effect has been found, but this may be inseparable from the induced euphoria. It is not in ordinary use as an antiemetic in cytostatic therapy.

Treatment of Nausea Due to Opioids

About 20% of patients treated with opioids suffer from nausea caused by the drug. The frequency of the nausea does not vary much according to the drug used, but none of the newer drugs have been shown to provoke less nausea than morphine. This type of nausea may have several causes:

Reduced gastric emptying because of reduced peristalsis.
Action on the chemoreceptor trigger zone.
Action on the vestibular system, causing nausea on movement (this action
    may also be due to postural hypotension induced by the drug).
Taste of the opioid mixture.
An effect of opioid-induced constipation.

Because nausea is more frequent in ambulant patients, it may be wise to administer a prophylactic antiemetic at the start of opioid therapy and then discontinue it after a few days. A majority of patients manage to take opioids without antiemetics for long periods. In bedridden patients nausea is less frequent. Since patients should be sedated as little as possible, the drug of choice against opioid nausea would be a high-potency neuroleptic and/or metoclopramide. The latter is very effective in the proper dosage, especially if the major cause of nausea is gastric stasis, but the effect does not last long. It needs to be taken half an hour before the opioid to achieve the best effect. The advantage of high-potency neuroleptics is the long duration of action, so that they need to be taken only one to three times a day.

Haloperidol, 0.5–2.0 mg in the morning, afternoon, and evening, usually has a good effect without too many side effects, and the lower doses are usually enough. With some patients it can be administered once a day, 1–5 mg at night. Alternatives are prochlorperazine, 5–10 mg × 2–3, or perphenazine, 2–4 mg × 3–4. Metoclopramide combines well with high-potency neuroleptics, even though this increases the risk of extrapyramidal side effects. These, however, are rare and usually present no problem.

Nausea caused by opioid intake should not normally be treated with propylamino-phenothiazine neuroleptics (chlorpromazine and related drugs) during the day, because these drugs have a strongly sedative effect which, combined with the sedative effect of the opioid, will put many patients practically out of action. They do not combine well with metoclopramide either, because they counteract the latter's stimulating effect on the gastrointestinal tract. In the evening, however, a low-potency neuroleptic can provide both an antiemetic and a sedative effect, and a good choice would be chlorpromazine, 10–50 mg, 1 to 2 hours before bedtime.

If the drugs mentioned above are not effective, an antihistamine can be tried, either alone or in combination with a high-potency neuroleptic/metoclopramide. A good choice is hydroxyzine, 10–25 mg × 2–4, or cyclizine, 50 mg × 1–3; meclozine, 25–50 mg × 1–2; or the more sedative promethazine, 25–50 mg in the evening.

If none of these drugs has the desired effect, glucocorticosteroids can be given in addition, since they may have a good effect on nausea from opioids. The usual dose is 10–30 mg of prednisolone per day or a corresponding amount of another drug (see Table 4). Sometimes higher doses may be used.

Treatment of Nausea Caused by Peripherally Acting Analgesics

Most peripherally acting analgesics have a local erosive effect on the stomach. They also weaken the mucous barrier, possibly due to their inhibition of prostaglandin synthesis, since prostaglandins may help to strengthen the mucous barrier of the stomach. These ulcerogenic effects can cause considerable nausea and vomiting. Gastrointestinal side effects can be an indication that the patient will develop gastrointestinal bleeding unless the drug is discontinued. If, however, there are strong indications for continuing with the analgesic, *enterosoluble alternatives* should be tried or a different NSAID with a lower frequency of side effects (diflunisal or sulindac) should be substituted. The ulcerogenic effect may be inhibited by *histamine H₂ blockers* such as cimetidine or ranitidine. Cimetidine very occasionally interacts with opioids and makes the patient very sedated or provokes hallucinations. *Sucralfate* reduces the gastric irritation caused by prostaglandin synthesis inhibitors. It binds to the lining of the stomach and gives local protection against the gastric acid. It also has a certain stimulating effect on prostaglandin synthesis. The action is entirely local and very little is absorbed, so it has very few side effects. Antacids may also be used together with an NSAID, but this often reduces the bioavailability of the drug. Recently, misoprostol (a prostaglandin analog) has been introduced for the treatment of NSAID-induced ulcers. This compound has proven very effective, but its use may be limited by side effects, for example, diarrhea.

Treatment of Nausea Caused by Cytostatic Therapy

Patients undergoing cytostatic therapy often suffer badly from nausea and vomiting. The nausea is usually worst during and just after the course of treatment, but some patients feel sick for days afterward and often have to be treated by their general physician. Many people develop a conditioned reflex to the treatment, and if they experienced nausea during the first course, it often becomes worse each time, until they start vomiting at the mere thought of a hospital.

Nausea and vomiting depend on the type and dose of cytostatic. Cisplatin, doxorubicin, dacarbazine, chlormethine, and iphosphamide are all strongly emetic in high doses. Cyclophosphamide, dactinomycin, 5-fluorouracil, mitomycin, and high-dose methotrexate are moderately emetic, and the VINCA alkaloids and low doses of methotrexate and bleomycin have little emetic effect.

Nausea should be prevented as far as possible by administering effective doses of antiemetics right from the beginning of the first course of treatment. This will reduce the nausea in subsequent treatments. It is very important and also easier to prevent nausea from occurring than to treat nausea that has already begun.

When the cytostatic is one that usually provokes moderate nausea, metoclopramide is a good choice. The usual dose is 20 mg orally or rectally before the treatment starts, followed by a new dose every 2 to 3 hours. Sometimes the drug is given as a continuous infusion. A number of recent studies have investigated the effect of the infusion of high doses of metoclopramide, 1–3 mg/kg, every 2 hours. A good anti-emetic effect was observed, but sedation was found to increase somewhat, and occasionally acute dystonia occurred, especially in patients under the age of 30. The antiemetic effect can be increased by combining metoclopramide with corticosteroids. A well-tried regimen is to give 8 mg of dexamethasone orally before the treatment starts, followed by 4–8 mg every 4 hours. Methylprednisolone, 250 mg × 4, has also been shown to have a good effect.

High-potency neuroleptics such as haloperidol, droperidol, and prochlorperazine have also been shown to alleviate nausea in doses well below those used in psychiatric conditions. The combination of high-potency neuroleptics and metoclopramide increases the antiemetic effect, but at the risk of acute dystonia, even though this rarely occurs. If it should do so, biperiden, 5–10 mg, should be administered intramuscularly or slowly intravenously.

If the patient needs to be sedated during the treatment, low-potency neuroleptics are used, such as chlorpromazine, 25–250 mg orally or parenterally two to four times a day. The patient becomes strongly sedated with the higher doses, but this may be an advantage because it causes a certain amount of amnesia, which helps to counteract the development of a conditioned reflex to the cytostatic treatment.

An additive antiemetic effect to metoclopramide, high-potency neuroleptics, or steroids can be achieved by administering antihistamines as well, such as difenhydramine, 50 mg intramuscularly. Diazepam, 5–20 mg before treatment, can also help to reduce anxiety and conditioned reflexes. Tetrahydrocannabinol has been shown to alleviate nausea, but the feeling of inebriation it induces puts many patients off.

ANOREXIA AND CACHEXIA

Cancer patients very often (in more than two-thirds of cases) suffer from anorexia (diminished appetite), leading to oligophagia (diminished intake of food). Anorexia has a large number of causes, among them:

Unappetizing food.
Problems affecting the mouth.
Pain.
Nausea.
Hypercalcemia, hyponatremia, uremia.
Altered sense of taste due to cancer.
Medication: analgesics, cytostatics, hormones, digitalis.
Radiotherapy.
Constipation.
Anxiety and depression.
Idiopathic.

Laboratory animals with some types of implanted cancer spontaneously reduce their food intake, but the pathogenesis of this form of anorexia is not clear. It is probably due to humoral factors secreted from the tumor. These factors may be sympathicomimetic, since some beta-adrenergic drugs (e.g., amphetamines) reduce the appetite. They may also be biogenic amines such as tryptophan or serotonin, which are transported to the hypothalamus and induce anorexia in this way. High levels of glucose and lactic acid in the blood, found in some cancer patients, may also contribute to anorexia.

Many cancer patients have an altered sense of taste and smell and often prefer sweeter, colder, and spicier food than they used to, and generally not food that contains a lot of urea (meat). Some patients say that their sense of taste disappears almost completely.

Food therefore needs to be presented in an appetizing and attractive way and in small portions. Some patients' appetites are improved if an alcoholic drink is served before and during the meal. The atmosphere at mealtimes is also important—there should be plenty of time, and many people prefer to have their meals in company rather than alone. Anorexia can be symptomatically treated with *glucocorticosteroids*, such as prednisolone, 5–30 mg per day, or dexamethasone, 2–4 mg per day. The appetite usually returns within about a week, and the sense of taste is also improved. If there is no effect after 2 weeks, however, the treatment can be discontinued. Tricyclic antidepressants (amitriptyline) also increase the appetite in some cases. Anabolic steroids can be tried.

Cachexia with emaciation, which is common in cancer patients, cannot be explained only by the reduced intake of food and the increased loss of protein. Cancer also causes metabolic changes. One of these is increased gluconeogenesis, a process requiring a great deal of energy as it converts fat and protein to glucose. Much of the glucose is consumed by the tumor, which breaks it down anaerobically, so that the energy is not utilized properly. It has recently been found that the body produces a substance called cachectin (also known as tumor necrosis factor). The production of cachectin is greatly increased in some diseases, including cancer and infectious diseases, and contributed to the emaciation often seen in these conditions.

Intensive nutrition of cancer patients has been tried—for example, by feeding energy-rich nourishment through a nasogastric catheter. This prevents weight loss and increases the patient's well-being for some time. It is possible that the increased energy supply benefits the tumor growth as well, but even so the improved condition will enable the patient to tolerate cytostatic or radiotherapy and other forms of treatment better. Hyperalimentation has no effect in advanced cachexia, however.

Patients with cachexia can easily develop bedsores on bony protuberances because of their diminishing subcutaneous fat and the accompanying muscular atrophy, and measures must be taken to prevent this.

CONSTIPATION

Constipation in cancer patients can be caused by:

Inactivity.
A diet poor in fiber.

Too little liquid, dehydration.
Side effects of medication, especially opioids and drugs with an anticho-
    linergic effect.
Biochemical disturbances: hypercalcemia, hypokalemia.
Intestinal tumor or peritoneal metastases.
Paraplegia.
Advanced disease with pronounced weakness.

Stomach pains are often due to constipation. If this is not recognized, and
the dose of opioid is increased, the symptoms will be aggravated rather
than alleviated. Because constipation is so common in cancer patients, it
should be prevented before it has a chance to become a problem. When
possible, patients should be encouraged to increase their activity, their
intake of fiber, and the amount of liquid they drink. All patients who take
opioids should be given laxatives prophylactically from the first day. If this
is not done, they can become so intractably constipated that it causes more
problems than the pain itself. Opioids inhibit peristalsis, so the most rational treatment is an agent that stimulates peristalsis—like casanthranol,
senna, cascara, bisacodyl, and so forth. This should be combined with an
agent that softens and increases the volume of the stools. A commonly
used compound drug is Peri-Colace, 1 capsule one to four times a day. If
this is not effective, lactulose can also be given, in doses of 10–30 ml per
day, two to three times a day. Stimulation of the peristalsis sometimes
causes colic, especially in patients who have previously suffered from "irritable colon," and lactulose can provoke meteorism, especially at first.
    Neostigmine sometimes has to be given in cases of paraplegia to
initiate intestinal function.

DIARRHEA

Diarrhea may be caused by:

Obstructive conditions: tumor with incomplete intestinal obstruction,
    long-lasting constipation.
Steatorrhea: pancreatic insufficiency (tumor), bile duct obstruction, liver
    failure, bacterially induced malabsorption.
Side effects of the treatment: broad-spectrum antibiotics, cytostatics, laxa-
    tives, abdominal radiotherapy.
Medullary thyroid carcinoma.
Functional intestinal disease.
Gastroenteritis.
Mental stress.

The obstructive conditions should be treated causally if possible. Rectal
exploration should always be done in cases of diarrhea to exclude severe
fecal impaction.
    Surgery should be considered in cases of steatorrhea. Symptomatic

treatment consists of administering tablets or granules containing pancreatic enzymes and, if necessary, bile acid. It is important to impress on the patient that the preparation has to be taken before *every* meal.

The patient's food should contain as little fat as possible. Medium-chain triglyceride (MCT) oil can be given in difficult cases, since it is easily absorbed even when there is insufficient bile and lipase in the intestines.

Bacterially induced malabsorption is diagnosed by a probe into the small intestine and a microbiological investigation. This is an unpleasant procedure, and if the diagnosis is suspected it is worth trying to treat the condition first with tetracycline, 250 mg four times a day for 2 to 3 weeks, or metronidazole, 200 mg four times a day.

Diarrhea caused by broad-spectrum antibiotics of cytostatics usually stops when the medication is discontinued. After radiotherapy, however, it can continue for a long time and actually become worse. Diarrhea caused by medullary thyroid carcinoma is probably due to increased production of prostaglandins in the intestine.

The most commonly used drugs are codeine, diphenoxylate combined with atropine, and loperamide. Codeine, 25–50 mg three to four times a day, can be used if an analgesic is needed as well. Diphenoxylate is a centrally acting analgesic that belongs to the morphine group but has no strong analgesic effect. The atropine component causes dryness of the mouth. The usual dose is one to two tablets three to four times a day, but it should not be given to patients with reduced liver function. Loperamide has no effect on the central nervous system and little anticholinergic effect. The patient should start with one to two tablets a day and increase gradually if necessary; up to eight tablets a day can be taken. Morphine or methadone taken to relieve pain will also provide symptomatic relief of the diarrhea. Diarrhea caused by medullary thyroid carcinoma should be treated with drugs that inhibit prostaglandin synthesis (NSAIDs).

GASTROINTESTINAL OBSTRUCTIONS

Gastrointestinal obstruction may be caused by:

Benign lesion
Adhesions
Primary neoplasm
Secondary neoplasm
Massive constipation
Terminal disease

Colorectal cancer and cancer of the cervix and ovary are the neoplasms most commonly associated with gastrointestinal obstruction. The patient has increasing distension of the abdomen, abdominal discomfort and pain, severe constipation and often no flatus, and nausea and vomiting. The bowel sounds may be high-pitched, but this is not always the case.

Some patients have overflow diarrhea. X-rays reveal distended loops of bowel; in some cases a radiodiagnostic small bowel enema may be needed. The patient's pain is most often a continuous, deep, aching visceral pain with referred pain to superficial areas in addition to bouts of colic.

Surgery should always be considered and is often the treatment of choice even in patients with far advanced cancer. It is, however, possible to gain control over the pain and vomiting for several weeks or months without surgery, and surgery should therefore be employed only if there is a fairly good chance of improved quality of life after the operation.

The use of intravenous fluid and nasogastric tube is of limited value. It should be used only in patients waiting for surgery and in patients who are likely to improve fairly quickly. It is not justified to use this method for prolonged treatment, because it is often uncomfortable for the patient and may even aggravate the condition (see p. 180).

The main symptoms to control are pain and vomiting. The deep aching pains respond well to opioids. Many patients are able to take morphine by mouth. If this is not possible, the opioid can be given by continuous subcutaneous infusion. If the patient is unable to take peroral medication, an anticholinergic can be administered by continuous subcutaneous infusion. Commonly used is scopolamine, 0.3–2.0 mg/24 hours. This relieves colic by reducing the peristalsis. It also has an antiemetic effect and diminishes secretion of saliva, which may be an advantage in nauseated patients. The sedation induced by the drug may be beneficial to some patients but rather distressing to others.

The nausea is treated preferably with a high-potency neuroleptic like haloperidol, 1–5 mg per 24 hours in one to three doses, or the antihistaminic drug cyclizine, 50 mg two or three times daily. These drugs may be administered by mouth or by continuous subcutaneous infusion. Scopolamine may be given together with one of these drugs to augment the antiemetic effect.

It is important to advise the patient to eat small meals and to eat early in the day. There is no need to force the patient to drink or to give intravenous fluid, as this is usually not beneficial for the patient (see p. 180).

HICCUPS

Patients with a tumor in the mediastinum or upper abdomen or with uremia may suffer from long bouts of hiccups.

The hiccups may respond well to chlorpromazine, 10–25 mg every 4 to 8 hours as needed, or metoclopramide, 10–20 mg three to six times a day. Swallowing a viscous liquid containing lidocaine may stop the hiccups. A subcutaneous injection of ephedrine, 10–25 mg, may be effective.

If the hiccups prove intractable, a block of the phrenic nerve can be considered. The effectiveness of this operation must be weighed against the resulting reduced respiratory capacity caused by paresis of the diaphragm.

SYMPTOMS FROM THE UROGENITAL TRACT

The muscles of the urinary bladder consist of the sphincter and the muscles in the bladder wall (detrusor muscles). When the latter contract the urine is expelled. The urinary bladder has a dual nerve supply: sympathetic nerves from the lumbar sympathetic trunk secrete norepinephrine, which contracts the sphincter and relaxes the detrusor muscle. Acetylcholine from parasympathetic nerves S2–S4 has the opposite effect. The bladder muscles are thus affected by drugs mimicking the action of the sympathetic/parasympathetic nervous system. Prostaglandins increase the sensitivity of these muscles to stimulation, and aspirinlike drugs thus reduce this sensitivity. Opioids increase the tone in both sphincter and detrusor muscles. This does not usually cause any problems, although a few patients have difficulties in emptying the bladder, and some develop symptoms of urgency incontinence.

URINARY INCONTINENCE, URINE RETENTION, AND URINARY TRACT INFECTIONS

The treatment of these conditions in cancer patients is more or less the same as in general medicine and will therefore not be dealt with here in any detail. Permanent catheters can be freely used in patients with a short life expectancy since this makes care of the patient easier for the patient, the nursing staff, and the family. When the catheter has been inserted under the most sterile conditions possible, a urinary tract antiseptic should be given prophylactically, such as methenamine hippurate, 1 g twice a day. This can be taken in tablet form or as a soluble powder. The pH of the urine must be checked during the treatment, because the drug depends on acidic urine for its effect. Vitamin C or ammonium chloride can be used to increase the acidity. Manifest symptoms of infection should be treated with a complete antibiotic cure and, if necessary, repeated instillations of chlorhexidine.

BLADDER SPASMS

Spasms of the bladder or urethral muscles may be caused by:

Irritation due to local tumor growth.
Radiotherapy or cytostatic therapy.
Cystitis.
Irritation from a permanent catheter.

Causal treatment should be given if possible. If the pain is due to the catheter, rinsing of the bladder can be tried, or manipulation or changing of the catheter. Drugs that reduce the detrusor activity are primarily anticholinergics that act mainly on the urinary tract, for example, flavoxantine chloride, 200 mg four times a day (if necessary up to 1200 mg per day), or phenazopyridine, 100–200 mg three times a day (can be increased to twice the dose or more if necessary). These drugs often give very good pain relief. Sometimes an NSAID, such as 250–500 mg naproxen in the morning and evening, is effective.

Bladder spasms usually do not respond well to opioids but it is often necessary to try them on such indications.

If the spasms do not respond to medication it may be necessary to block the sympathetic trunk at the lumbar level. An epidural catheter with a local anesthetic also blocks the sympathetic trunk.

SYMPTOMS FROM THE RESPIRATORY ORGANS

DYSPNEA

Local causes may be:

Tumors of the lung or mediastinum.
Lymphangitis carcinomatosa.
Pleural effusion (usually due to malignancy).
Atelectasis.
Pneumonia.
Obstructive or restrictive lung disease.
Lung fibrosis following radiotherapy or cytostatics (bleomycin).
Lung emboli.

Systemic causes may be:

Cardiac insufficiency (with lung edema).
Anemia.
Acidosis (due to uremia or diabetes).
Fever.
Emotional factors (anxiety).

Inoperable tumors that give rise to dyspnea are usually treatable with radiotherapy and/or cytostatics. If the dyspnea is progressing rapidly, large doses of steroids (e.g., dexamethasone, 4 mg four times a day) can give relief until the radio- or chemotherapy takes effect. Steroids can have a good symptomatic effect in lymphangitis carcinomatosa.

Pleural exudate should be drained if it causes discomfort, especially if the patient's condition is reasonably good. The instillation of a tetracycline derivative will lead to the formation of an interpleural fibrosis, and this can reduce the formation of fresh exudate. Patients in the terminal phase can be helped by methods other than draining, as described below.

If a cancer patient in poor condition develops *pneumonia*, it may be very difficult to decide whether to administer antibiotics. The patient's suffering, the prognosis, the patient's wishes, the family's attitude, and so on should be taken into consideration before deciding. If antibiotics are used, pivampicillin or trimethoprim-sulfamethoxazole is suitable.

The treatment of *anemia* by transfusion improves the patient's general condition and dyspnea and may allow the patient to tolerate active treatment better, to attend an important occasion, and so on. The effect of transfusion treatment, however, is usually short.

Symptomatic Treatment

When specific therapy no longer has any effect, the treatment must be concentrated on relieving the dyspnea, which is very distressing for patients, who feel as if they are being choked. The respiratory center is highly activated, and most patients are anxious and frightened, which aggravates the dyspnea. This vicious circle can be broken only if the patient can be calmed and assured of receiving effective treatment. Benzodiazepines are often useful here.

If the dyspnea is due to heart failure and lung edema, this can be treated along the usual lines by digitalis glycosides and diuretics. Theophyllamine should be given if there is an obvious obstruction. *Opioids* are the best medication for relieving the choking feeling and the anxiety. They reduce the respiratory frequency by decreasing the activity of the respiratory center, but this may improve the blood gas values because the reduced respiratory work demands less oxygen. Opioids should preferably be given orally—for instance, a morphine mixture where the dose can be varied according to the patient's symptoms, as in the case of pain. The usual starting dose is 5–20 mg × 6, and this can be increased as necessary. Relative contraindications to opioid therapy are chronic lung disease and respiratory insufficiency. As with pain, respiratory depression has not proved to be a problem with oral opioid therapy in doses appropriate to the patient's symptoms, and physicians with long experience of treating terminal cancer patients with dyspnea and asthma have observed few complications in oral opioid therapy.

If the dyspnea is very pronounced, the opioid has to be given intramuscularly or (preferably) intravenously, often in combination with a benzodiazepine. The risk of respiratory depression is greater in this situation, and the patient must be carefully followed up. This is not, however, a reason for not treating the patient, since dyspnea is extremely distressing and should be alleviated. A good method is to start with 10 mg of morphine intramuscularly or 5 mg intravenously and gradually increase the dose until the respiratory frequency reaches 12–20 per minute. Continuous intravenous infusion of morphine or subcutaneous infusion with a drug delivery pump can be very effective here. In case of an overdose, 0.1–0.4 mg of naloxone administered intravenously will rapidly reverse the effect of the opioid. But this is very seldom necessary.

Oxygen therapy can sometimes relieve dyspnea, usually in its more serious forms or in case of an acute aggravation. However, extra oxygen can provoke respiratory depression if the CO_2 is chronically elevated. Oxygen therapy should be used sparingly in chronic slight to moderate dyspnea because patients may easily become "addicted" to the oxygen and thus become less mobile than they would otherwise be. In terminal patients, being connected to an oxygen supply can be more unpleasant than comfortable because of the irritation from the nasal catheter or the mask.

COUGH

Coughing may be caused by irritation of any of the organs in the thorax— the pharynx, trachea, bronchi, pleura, pericardium, or diaphragm. It can be due to cigarette smoke or other irritating gases, to chronic obstructive lung disease, heart failure, lung infection, or mechanical irritation from an intrathoracic tumor. A third of all terminal cancer patients experience uncomfortable coughing, and so do the majority of patients with bronchogenic carcinoma.

Cough should be treated causally if possible. This may involve radiotherapy, cytostatic therapy, or occasionally surgery. In cases of manifest intrathoracic infection, antibiotics will relieve the cough, but in deciding whether to treat the infection the patient's total situation should be considered.

Usually coughing has to be treated *symptomatically*. It is important to give the patient plenty of hot drinks. Expectorants and mucolytics usually have little effect. Cough due to a tumor in the airways can be difficult to treat, even with the help of opium alkaloids or derivatives. Codeine, ethylmorphine, hydrocodone, and the commonest strong analgesics except for meperidine all have an antitussive effect, although higher than standard doses are usually necessary.

SYMPTOMS FROM THE SKIN

ULCERATING TUMORS

Ulcerating tumors can be painful and may smell very unpleasant owing to infection. The secretions may cause problems and they can bleed severely.

Radiotherapy or cytostatic treatment should be given if possible, and sometimes surgery is called for. All these treatments can considerably reduce the tumor size and provide a covering of skin.

If such treatment is impossible, wet compresses should be applied and changed frequently (two to four times a day). If the sore is "clean," a physiological saline solution should be used. If it is infected the compresses should be soaked in potassium permanganate solution or some other antiseptic. Local antibiotics should not be used. When the compresses are changed the lesion should be washed with chlorhexidine or hydrogen peroxide. Necrotic areas must be carefully excised. If there is necrosis, preparations containing proteolytic enzymes should be avoided because they can cause the delicate tissue to bleed. If, in spite of these precautions, the ulcer becomes severely infected or smells bad, antibiotics can be given orally after tissue culture and determination of the bacterial resistance. If the resistance cannot be determined, a broad-spectrum antibiotic can be given combined with a chemotherapeutic agent against anaerobic bacteria, which are frequently found in the ulcers. Fungal infection is also common and should be dealt with by a local antimycotic.

Spongostan or compresses soaked in an epinephrine solution should be used if there is persistent capillary bleeding. This can be topped by a pressure bandage if necessary. Cautious electrocoagulation can also be tried.

Pain can be helped by soaking the compresses in a solution of local anesthetic.

Acute severe bleeding may make the patient panic, and an intravenous injection of diazepam, 5–20 mg, or scopolamine, 0.3–0.6 mg, will calm the patient and induce a certain amnesia.

PRURITUS

Pruritus can be caused by local conditions such as dry skin, local allergic reactions, local infection by fungus and/or bacteria, or a reaction to soap, perfume, or a local ointment or cream. Dry skin can be treated with a moisturizing cream, water-resistant ointment, or oil, but not liniment, since this dries out the skin even more. Crotamiton cream is a local antipruritic. Cream containing a glucocorticosteroid should be used on inflamed skin, as long as the inflammation is not due to bacteria or fungi.

The commonest analgesics, including both opioids and NSAIDs (peripherally acting analgesics), can cause rashes and itching, and so do antibiotics. The laxative danthron occasionally causes itching.

Obstructive icterus (usually due to cancer of the pancreas or bile ducts) can provoke severe, almost unbearable itching. Surgical drainage should be carried out if possible. Cholestyramine binds the bile acid in the intestine and inhibits the enterohepatic circulation, so that the body loses bile acid. This can reduce the itching, but cholestyramine can of course only be used in cases of incomplete bile duct obstruction. The dose is 4 g dissolved in a solution and administered twice a day.

Some patients find that the drug gives them unpleasant side effects like diarrhea or constipation, and the treatment is difficult to carry out in terminal patients. Other forms of cancer, such as Hodgkin's disease, may be accompanied by pruritus, and pruritus frequently occurs in connection with renal insufficiency.

Antihistamines are generally used for the systemic treatment of pruritus. Commonly used drugs are hydroxyzine, 10–25 mg two to three times a day, dexchlorpheniramine, 2 mg two to four times a day, or other similar antihistamines. Promethazine, 10–50 mg, is both antipruritic and sedative and is thus a good preparation for use at night. Itching can also be soothed by systemic glucocorticosteroids, such as prednisolone tablets, 5–20 mg one to three times a day, which can be combined with antihistamines. Amitriptyline also helps in many types of pruritus.

SYMPTOMS WITH SYSTEMIC ETIOLOGY

DEHYDRATION

Dehydration in cancer patients is usually due to insufficient fluid intake, either because of nausea and vomiting or because of advanced disease and extreme weakness. If fluid is lost by vomiting it should be replaced intravenously, in order to reestablish the fluid balance and to rest the gastrointestinal tract and relieve the nausea.

Dehydration is commonly believed to be very distressing, but a good deal of clinical evidence suggests that the only unpleasant symptoms are dry mouth and throat. If these are treated locally by frequent moistening, supplemented by artificial saliva if necessary, patients rarely feel thirsty and therefore seldom need treatment with intravenous infusion or a nasogastric catheter. Dehydration may even have a beneficial effect, since it results in the reduction of all secretions. Thus, in gastrointestinal obstruction vomiting may be lessened, in pneumonia and pulmonary edema coughing and breathlessness may be reduced, and so on. Intravenous treatment is almost never used at hospices, which specialize in care of the dying, because it is not necessary to relieve the symptoms of dehydration and may even aggravate the patient's condition.

HYPERCALCEMIA

Hypercalcemia occurs in 40% of patients with multiple myeloma, in 30% with cancer of the breast with metastasis, in 13% with cancer of the kidney, and in just under 10% with other malignant diseases. It is usually due to osteolytic metastases. Ectopic hormone production will occasionally give rise to pseudohyperparathyroidism.

When the calcium level in serum is determined, the albumin values must be taken into consideration because about 50% of the calcium is bound to albumin and is thus inactive. At lower albumin concentrations the active fraction increases. The following formulas are commonly used:

Corrected calcium (mg/100 ml)

= measured calcium + 0.8[4 − measured albumin (g/100 ml)]   (U.S.)

or

Corrected calcium (mmol/l)

= measured calcium + 0.02 [40 − measured albumin (g/l)]   (U.K.)

A better method is to measure the ionized calcium if this is possible.

The symptoms of hypercalcemia are many and can be divided into four
    groups:
Neurological: tiredness, lethargy, apathy or more serious degrees of dis-
    turbed consciousness, muscular weakness, confusion, or psychosis.
Gastrointestinal: anorexia, nausea, vomiting, constipation, abdominal pain.
Renal: polyuria, polydipsia, kidney insufficiency.
Cardiovascular: arrhythmia, increased sensitivity to digitalis, hypertension.

Hypercalcemia can probably give rise to diffuse pain and reduce the pain-
relieving effect of opioids.
    Moderate hypercalcemia can be treated primarily by increasing the
fluid intake and taking a loop diuretic such as furosemide, 40–120 mg per
day. Thiazides should not be used with moderate hypercalcemia because
they reduce the elimination of calcium via the kidneys. The patient should
be encouraged to be as mobile as possible. Glucocorticosteroids should
also be given, for example, prednisolone, 20–100 mg per day, in decreasing doses until the lowest possible maintenance dose is reached. It usually
takes 3 to 5 days before the response to this treatment can be evaluated
and it works in less than 50% of patients. This treatment also relieves pain
in skeletal metastasis. In addition to the medication, calcium-containing
foods like milk and milk products should be avoided. If the hypercalcemia
persists, 1–3 g of cellulose phosphate powder or tablets can be given at
every meal, which will bind the calcium in the stomach and intestinal
secretions. The side effects are nausea and diarrhea, so many patients find
it unsatisfactory.
    Some patients have lower calcium levels after taking NSAIDs in ordi-
nary therapeutic doses. This treatment is worth trying when the hypercalcemia is accompanied by skeletal metastasis because it also has a good
effect on pain relief, but it is difficult to predict which patients will benefit
from it.
    If the treatment is not effective, it can be replaced by subcutaneous
administration of synthetic calcitonin, which the patient can easily learn to
carry out. Calcitonin prevents bone resorption and thus has a certain pain-
killing effect. The usual dose is 1 ml per day. The effect on serum calcium
is usually rapid, but continuous treatment is needed and this sometimes
causes the effect to diminish, so that the calcium level may rise again.
    A new and interesting therapeutic alternative consists of the diphos-
phonates clodronate and ethitronate, which prevent bone resorption probably by inhibiting osteoclast function and thereby osteolysis. The treat-

ment can be carried out orally, and there are few side effects. It relieves skeletal pain, and some studies even indicate that it may prolong the life of patients with breast cancer.

Mithramycin, which is a cytostatic, is necessary if the hypercalcemia is severe. Only one-tenth of the dose used in cytostatic therapy is used for hypercalcemia, and the side effects are correspondingly fewer, although bone marrow suppression may occur. The treatment is more intensive, requiring intravenous administration, and has to be carried out in a hospital. It is accompanied by furosemide and 2–4 l of intravenous physiological saline solution. This method usually has a good and rapid effect on hypercalcemia.

12

Treatment of Pain and Other Symptoms During the Last Few Days Before Death

Most people die in institutions. A patient who has been at home for most of the illness, however, should be able to die there, both for the patient's sake and that of the family. In this situation the family requires a good deal of information and practical help, so that they know what is likely to happen and what to do. Good contact with the family physician and a visiting nurse is therefore essential. Sudden hospitalization 1 or 2 days before death is not a good solution for the patient, who will be surrounded by strange doctors and nurses; even if the family is present at the end, the change of environment is a great strain at this time and can make a patient confused and insecure. In saying this I do not mean to instill a sense of guilt in people who are unable to care for a patient at home and need to use the services of an institution. I simply mean that where possible the primary health service should provide the necessary support and practical help to enable a patient to die in dignity in familiar surroundings.

TREATMENT OF PAIN

Many patients are able to continue with oral treatment until the last couple of days before death, and some right up to the end.

If a patient can no longer take medication orally, it must be given parenterally. Suppositories are an alternative but the absorption is slow and the effect varies. The uncertain mode of action makes them unsuitable for use in this phase, where the right dose has to be found quickly.

Morphine, hydromorphone, or heroin should be used for injections; methadone causes local irritation, especially when given intravenously. During the changeover to parenteral morphine therapy, 50–70% of the oral methadone dose or 25–50% of the oral morphine dose is given as a starting dose. The hydromorphone dose is usually one-fifth of this. Because of the great variations in bioavailability with oral treatment, the exact parenteral dose can be difficult to establish. It requires continual reevaluation of the effects to find the right dose rapidly. Many patients need smaller doses of an analgesic in the terminal phase than they did previously. If a patient has been taking opioids for some time, they must *not* be discontinued, even if the patient loses consciousness; otherwise the patient will develop abstinence symptoms and become very disturbed.

When analgesics have to be given parenterally during the last days of life, the best method is to give a continuous subcutaneous/intramuscular infusion by means of a drug delivery pump. Injections of morphine or hydromorphone every 4 hours are an alternative, but with this method the pain relief is more uneven. With intravenous infusion of morphine the daily dose can be given in 500 ml of saline solution. The starting dose is 5 mg intravenously and the rate of infusion is adjusted to the patient's pain and sedation. There is a risk of respiratory depression with this method, but in practice it is rarely a problem.

TREATMENT OF TERMINAL LUNG EDEMA AND THE DEATH RATTLE

Dyspnea and bubbling in the throat (the "death rattle") caused by extra amounts of fluid and mucous that the patient is unable to cough up can be unpleasant. The death rattle often frightens the other family members, who may take it as a sign that the patient is choking and suffering.

Dyspnea caused by lung edema can be effectively relieved by morphine, which should preferably be given as a continuous subcutaneous infusion with a drug delivery pump or, if this is not possible, by intramuscular injections or continuous intravenous infusion. The patient should preferably not be given large amounts of fluid during the last few days, since this can prolong the dying process and increase bronchial secretion, and it is not necessary to relieve thirst (see p. 00). The size of the morphine dose should be adjusted according to the degree of dyspnea (see p. 00). Oxygen can also relieve dyspnea, but a nasal catheter or a mask is often uncomfortable rather than soothing.

Belladonna alkaloids dry out the upper respiratory passages and thus counteract the rattling. Scopolamine (0.3–0.6 mg every 2 to 6 hours) is the best choice, since it has a sedative as well as a drying effect, although a few patients become excited instead. This can be counteracted by giving them physostigmine. Atropine, 0.3–1.0 mg, can also be tried, but it does have an excitatory effect. These drugs work best if given fairly early, before the rattling has become pronounced, because if it has been going on for a long time so much fluid has often accumulated in the bronchi and lungs that the drugs are of little use, their function being to prevent fresh secretion rather than dry up what is already there.

Some patients develop edema in the lower parts of the body (the backs of the thighs, over the sacrum and the lumbar vertebrae) during the last day. These parts of the body must be avoided when giving injections, since the drug will not be absorbed and therefore has no effect.

The combination of morphine and scopolamine or atropine provides effective relief during the last few hours and helps to make the dying process pass peacefully.

Appendix

APPENDIX: Medications Used in the Treatment of Pain

U.S. approved name	U.S. trade name
Acetaminophen	Acephen, Anuphen, Suppap, Ty-Pap, Neopap, Anacin, Genapap, Panadol, Tempra, Tylenol, Pedric, Phenaphen, A'Cenol, Aceta, Actamin, Aspirin Free Pain Relief, Conacetol, Dapa, Gerebs, Halenol, Meda Tab, Panex, Topar, Tenol, Ty-tabs, Valadol, Valorin, Ty-Caps
Amitriptyline	Saroten
Aspirin	Easprin, Zorprin, numerous otc*
Atropine	Dey-Dose
Bisacodyl	Dacodyl, Dulcolax, Bisco-Lax
Bupivacaine	Sensoricaine, Marcaine
Buprenorfin	Temgesic, Buprenex
Butorphanol	Stadol
Carbamazepine	Tegretol, Epitol
Casanthranol	Cantralax, Peristim
Cascara	Cascara Sagrada (various)
Chlorimipramine	(Clomipramine)
Clotrimazole	Mycelex, Gyne-Lotrimin, Lotrimin
Codeine	Codeine sulfate, Codeine phosphate
Cyclizine	Marezine
Danthron	
Diflunisal	Dolobid
Doxorubicin	Adriamycin
Fenbufen	
Fenoprofen	
Flavoxantine	Urispas
Flupentixol	
Fluphenazine	Permitil, Prolixin
Flurbiprofen	Ansaid, Froben
Furosemide	Fumide, Lasix, Luramide
Haloperidol	Haldol,Haloperidol
Heroin	
Hydromorphone	Dilaudid
Hydroxyzine	Atarax, Atozine, Durrax, Anxanil, Hy-Pam, Vamate, Vistaril, E-Vista, Hydroxacen, Hyzine-50, Quiess, Vistacon, Vistaject, Vistaquel
Ibuprofen	Aches-N-Pain, Advil, Haltram, Ibuprin, Medipren, Midol, Nuprin, Pamprin-IB, Trendar, Motrin, Ifen, Rufen
Indomethacin	Indameth, Indocin, Indo-Lemmon
Ketoconazole	Nizoral
Ketoprofen	Orudis
Lactulose	Duphalac, Cephulac, Cholac, Constilac, Chronulac
Levorphanol	Levo-Dromoran
Loperamide	Imodium
Meclizone	Antivert, Antrizine, Ru-Vert-M, Wehvert, Bonine, Dizmiss, Motion Cure
Meperidine	Demerol
Methadone	Dolophine
Methenamine hippurate	Hiprex, Urex
N/A	
N/A	
Morphine	
Immediate release	Astramorph, Duramorph, MSIR, Roxmol, RMS
Slow release	MS Contin, Roxanol
Nalbuphine	Nubain
Naproxen	Anaprox, Naprosyn
Nortriptyline	Aventyl HCl, Pamelor
Pentazocine	Talwin
Perphenazine	Trilafon

British approved name	British trade name
Paracetamol	
Frusemide	
Diamorphine	
Pethidine	
Methotrimeprazine	
Mianserin	Bolvidon, Tolvon

U.S. approved name	U.S. Trade name
Phenazopyridine	Tyridium, Azo-Standard, Bardium, Di-Azo, Eridium, Geridium, Phenazodine, Pyridiate, Urodine, Urogesic
Piroxicam	Feldene
Plicamycin	Mithracin
Prochlorperazine	Compazine, Chlorpazine
Promethazine	Phenergan, Phenameth, Anergan, Prometh, Prorex
Propoxyphene chloride	Darvon Pulvules, Dolene, Doxaphene, Prophene
Propoxyphene napsylate	Darvon-N
Scopolamine	Transderm-Scōp,
Senna	Senexon, Senokot, Genna, Senna-Gen, Senolax, Gentlax, Black-Drought, Dr. Caldwell Senna Laxative, Fletcher's Castoria for Children
Sucralfate	Carafate
Sulindac	Clinoril
Tamoxifen	Nolvadex
Trazodone	Desyrel, Trialodine
Valproate	

*otc, over the counter.

British approved name	British trade name
Mithramycin	
	Prothazine, Phencen, V-Gan-25, K-Phen, Mallergan, Pentazine
Dextropropoxyphene-chloride	
Dextropropoxyphene-napsylate	
Hyoscine	

Index